CLEAR BODY

CLEAR MIND

THE EFFECTIVE PURIFICATION PROGRAM

CLEAR BODY CLEAR MIND

THE EFFECTIVE PURIFICATION PROGRAM

L. RON HUBBARD

Bridge

Publications, Inc.

A
HUBBARD®
PUBLICATION

Published in the USA by
BRIDGE PUBLICATIONS, INC.
4751 Fountain Avenue
Los Angeles, California 90029

ISBN 1-57318-224-9

Published in all other countries by
NEW ERA® PUBLICATIONS INTERNATIONAL ApS
Store Kongensgade 53
1264 Copenhagen K, Denmark

Important
Note

IN READING THIS BOOK, be very certain you never go past a word you do not fully understand.

The only reason a person gives up a study or becomes confused or unable to learn is because he or she has gone past a word that was not understood.

The confusion or inability to grasp or learn comes AFTER a word that the person did not have defined and understood.

Have you ever had the experience of coming to the end of a page and realizing you didn't know what you had read? Well, somewhere earlier on that page you went past a word that you had no definition for or an incorrect definition for.

Here's an example. "It was found that when the crepuscule arrived the children were quieter and when it was not present, they were much livelier." You see what happens. You think you don't understand the whole idea, but the inability to understand came entirely from the one word you could not define, *crepuscule,* which means twilight or darkness.

It may not only be the new and unusual words that you will have to look up. Some commonly used words can often be misdefined and so cause confusion.

This datum about not going past an undefined word is the most important fact in the whole subject of study. Every subject you have taken up and abandoned had its words which you failed to get defined.

Therefore, in studying this book be very, very certain you never go past a word you do not fully understand. If the material becomes confusing or you can't seem to grasp it, there will be a word just earlier that you have not understood. Don't go any further, but go back to BEFORE you got into trouble, find the misunderstood word and get it defined.

FOOTNOTES AND DEFINITIONS

To help you comprehend the material in this book, words that might be easily misunderstood are defined as footnotes the first time they appear in the text. Each word so defined has a small number to its right, and the definition appears at the bottom of the page beside the corresponding number.

Words sometimes have several meanings, but only the meaning of the word as it is used in the text is given in the footnote. Other definitions for the word can be found in a dictionary.

A glossary is also provided for you at the back of this book consisting of all the footnoted definitions. Beside each glossary definition you will find the chapter in which it appears and the footnote number so you can refer back to it if you wish.

INTRODUCTION

THE TWENTIETH CENTURY brought miraculous changes in technology and industry. Again and again, science refashioned or outwitted nature to improve our health and comfort. But as the years passed, a cloud gathered around this progress. Our environment—and our bodies—began to react to something new in man's history: a continuous assault of man-made drugs, toxins and radiation.

This assault is massive. With a multitude of synthetic chemicals in use and new chemicals introduced each day, there is no way to avoid exposure to toxins, pesticides, drug residues and chemicals that come to you in the food you eat, the water you drink and the air you breathe.

The magnitude of this problem cannot be overstated. In addition to ruining one's physical condition, the harmful effects of drugs and chemical residues reduce awareness and block any stable advancement to mental or spiritual well-being.

Drug abuse continues to be a huge problem across the planet, leaving no country or social stratum immune to its devastation. Besides drugs like heroin and opium that have existed for ages, new drugs are produced each year, chemically designed to produce strong, mind-altering effects. And these "designer" drugs can be even more potent than drugs like heroin, and their long-range effects remain unknown.

Air and water pollution bring harmful toxins to even the most remote corners of the globe. Man-made chemicals stored in the fat of seals poison native people in remote arctic areas. Significant traces of the insecticide DDT have been found in the tree bark of wild forests, hundreds of miles from any civilization, while pesticide residues taint breast milk throughout the world. The deterioration of the upper atmosphere by pollution has resulted in increased levels of ultraviolet radiation. When inadequate safeguards are applied, the use of nuclear power can pose serious health threats from radiation exposure (as at Chernobyl).

It is no longer a question of whether drugs and man-made toxins destroy life, but how much they will destroy and how soon.

In a very real sense, drugs and other man-made chemicals do not belong in the body. They dull the senses. They cause or contribute to a wide range of illnesses, from cancer and nerve damage to lowered immunity. Even exposures as innocuous as perfume can cause some individuals to experience severe reactions.

But it is the insidious nature of this problem which makes it most dangerous. Take for example the person who was involved with street drugs at an earlier age, stopped taking them, but still experiences their negative influences—even years later. Or the man who has unwittingly accumulated traces of dozens of pesticides and other toxic chemicals in his body, and now suffers from a wide range of illnesses and fatigue.

In the face of such an overwhelming barrage of toxins and drugs encountered on a daily basis, what can be done to free oneself from the devastating effects?

The answer came from the breakthrough discoveries of L. Ron Hubbard. In 1977, while researching the harmful effects drugs have on a person's spiritual advancement, he discovered that the drug LSD left residual deposits in the user's fatty tissue. He found that these residuals could continue to cause adverse reactions in these individuals months and even years after the original "trip" was over. He later extended his discoveries to other drugs and toxic compounds. He then developed and released a purification (detoxification) procedure that could safely reduce or eliminate the toxic chemicals accumulated in fatty tissues.

At the time, these were radical ideas. The idea that chemical residues stored for years in the fat was controversial. The idea that these residues could actually cause adverse effects was revolutionary. Nonetheless, the Purification program created dramatic effects on those who participated in it.

Research in subsequent years has validated Mr. Hubbard's theory, and has demonstrated the value of the program for a variety of toxic exposures. This work has shown beyond question that the Purification program described in this book, when followed exactly, can be remarkably effective. In fact, thousands upon thousands across the planet have freed themselves from the biochemical devastation caused by drugs and toxic substances.

As his intention was solely to clear the way for an individual's mental and spiritual progress, L. Ron Hubbard claimed no medical results for his work. However, the Purification program has extremely broad application—as all truly basic discoveries do.

In the course of clinical practice, it has been possible to observe firsthand the results of the Purification program. They have been nothing less than miraculous. These cases have included patients with minor effects of residual toxins, people who were exposed to toxic chemicals on the job, casual drug users and long-term heavy drug users with bodies ravaged from the effects of those drugs. The depression, hopelessness and fear which often accompany such problems were also evident in many of these patients. Upon completion of the Purification program, these people were changed, both physically and mentally.

The common theme expressed by people who have completed the program is that they are no longer encumbered by the chemicals which were shutting off their lives. They express increased mental clarity and new hope for the future. Upon completion of the program, their lives are happier, healthier and more productive.

Studies done over the decades provide repeated evidence of the program's effectiveness in eliminating toxins from the body. For example, consider the following:

• While monitoring the rehabilitation of cocaine and Valium addicts using the Purification program, a medical doctor and a molecular biologist found that previously undetectable drugs appeared in both the urine and sweat of former drug users. In other words, these residual drugs were dislodged as a result of the program and eliminated, freeing each individual from the harmful effects of these drugs.

• A young woman had spent six months on a job that required her to hose off the filters of an oil-burning generator. She had developed a variety of physical symptoms, accompanied by a general hopelessness about life. She was enrolled in a supervised Purification program. On the fourth day of the program, a blackish greasy material began to ooze out of the pores of her skin. This continued for several days and eventually ceased. When she completed the program, her physical complaints were gone. An even greater relief she expressed was the return of the mental and physical energy and alertness that we associate with good health.

• The deadly chemical dioxin found in the military defoliant "Agent Orange" and used during the Vietnam War, poisoned thousands that were exposed to it, including American servicemen. Years later a cardiologist conducted tests on a person who had been exposed to this chemical but subsequently completed the Purification program. He found that the patient's level of dioxin had reduced by 29 percent immediately after the program and an astounding 97 percent eight months later. And all previous symptoms attributed to this poisoning had disappeared.

• A number of military veterans who served in the Gulf War returned with various debilitating conditions. These individuals lived and fought in the presence of a long list of toxins, ranging from pesticides, the byproducts of oil well fires, radioactive shells and, possibly, chemical warfare agents. Several veterans suffering from this "Gulf War Syndrome" have completed this program. All have reported remarkable improvements.

In addition, L. Ron Hubbard also noticed that the program had great workability in reducing certain effects of exposure to harmful forms of radiation.

The Chernobyl disaster is considered one of the worst nuclear accidents ever to have occurred. Workers and residents were exposed to a wide range of radiation doses, along with great stress and anxiety. Many of these people are now suffering from a number of illnesses related to the event. While the specific relation of these illnesses to radiation is still the subject of scientific studies, an approach that would return these men, women and children to a state of good mental and physical health was needed.

Mr. Hubbard's program was applied to several Chernobyl-affected groups. In Kazakhstan, a group of men who worked on the repair and recovery from the Chernobyl disaster (known as "liquidators") had been suffering from these illnesses for several years, and had not responded to standard medical treatments. The men were placed on the Purification program, and all reported marked improvement from the debilitating conditions from which they had suffered. In another group who lived in one of the most radioactively contaminated regions of the Russian Federation, similar results were reported—including clinical evidence that the men's immune systems had been revitalized by the program.

The ongoing utilization of the Purification program, in many quarters, has been documented in scientific papers published by various groups ranging from the World Health Organization's International Agency for Research on Cancer, and the Royal Swedish Academy of Sciences, to the United States Environmental Protection Agency.

These papers in turn have led to several international conferences and meetings, bringing together physicians, government officials, researchers, and drug rehabilitation specialists. They represent the only international attempts to consider drug abuse and environmental exposure as *related* problems—a notion that helps to explain the growing popularity of the Purification program.

The problem of preserving the well-being of individuals living in a toxic world has been begging for a solution. With this book, that solution is in your hands.

L. Ron Hubbard's Purification program remains the only proven and safe method for reducing or eliminating chemical residues from the body. It has been used to alleviate the symptoms and concerns of people exposed to radiation. With each year, the importance of this discovery to every man, woman and child on this planet becomes more evident.

This could be the most important book you will ever read.

David Root, M.D., M.P.H.
Board-Certified Occupational Medicine Specialist

James Barnes
Certified Health Physicist, Specialist in radioactivity and radiation safety

CLEAR BODY, CLEAR MIND

THE EFFECTIVE PURIFICATION PROGRAM

CONTENTS

PART 1: THE PURIFICATION PROGRAM: THEORY, PRINCIPLES & ELEMENTS

PART 2: THE PURIFICATION PROGRAM: GUIDELINES FOR SUCCESSFUL APPLICATION

APPENDIX:

THE PURIFICATION PROGRAM:

THEORY, PRINCIPLES & ELEMENTS

CHAPTER ONE

OUR BIOCHEMICAL SOCIETY

THE PLANET HAS HIT A BARRIER which prevents any widespread social progress—drugs and other biochemical substances.

These can put people into a condition which not only prohibits and destroys physical health but which can prevent any stable advancement in mental or spiritual well-being.

That's the situation today.

We live in a biochemical society.

Bio means "life; of living things." (It is from the Greek word *bios,* which means "life" or "way of life.")

Chemical means "of or having to do with chemicals." And chemicals are the substances, simple or complex, which are the building blocks of matter.

By *biochemical* is meant "the interaction of life forms and chemical substances."

Toxic substance is a term which has been used to describe drugs, chemicals, or any substance shown to be poisonous or harmful to an organism. The word *toxic* comes from the Greek word *toxikon* which originally meant a poison in which arrows were dipped.

The human body is made up of certain exact chemicals and chemical compounds, and complex chemical processes go on continuously within it. Some substances, such as nutrients, air and water, are vital to the continuation of these processes and for maintaining the body's health. Some substances are relatively neutral when entered into the body, causing neither benefit nor damage. *Toxic* substances are those which upset the body's normal chemical balance or interfere with its chemical processes. Some of them can wreak havoc, blocking or perverting vital body functions and making the body ill or even killing it.

Detoxification would be the action of removing a poison or a poisonous effect from something (such as from one's body).

TOXINS IN ABUNDANCE

There has been an enormous volume of material written on the subject of toxic substances, their reported effects and the prospects for their handling. Examples abound in publications and news reports.

Unfortunately, the current environment is becoming permeated with these life-hostile elements. Drugs, radioactive wastes, pollutants and chemical agents of various types are all a part of the scene and, apparently, more and more prevalent as time goes on.

According to studies, even some of the things that are put in a can of peas or a can of soup are to be considered toxic. They are preservatives and the action of a preservative is to impede decay. Yet digestion and cellular action are based on decay. In other words, those things might be great for the manufacturer as they preserve his product, *but* they could be very bad for the consumer. It is not that I am on a food faddism kick or a kick against preservatives; the point is that man is surrounded by toxins. This one example alone (preservatives in foods) is an example of the degree to which one can be confronted with toxic substances in the course of daily living.

And with the enemies of various countries using widespread drug addiction as a defeatist mechanism, with nations vying with each other in the manufacture and testing of nuclear weapons (and so increasing the amount of radioactive material free in the environment), with painkillers and sedatives so easily available and with the increased use of industrial and agricultural chemicals, to say nothing of the substances developed for chemical warfare, we face a growing problem.

Putting it quite bluntly, this society, at this time, is riddled with toxic substances.

To briefly point out certain data regarding those substances which pose a threat to individuals and to society at large will bring the biochemical situation more clearly into focus.

STREET DRUGS

Research has demonstrated that the single most destructive element present in our current culture is drugs.

The acceleration of widespread use of drugs such as LSD, heroin, cocaine, "angel dust," marijuana and a long list of others has contributed heavily to a debilitated society. Reportedly, some of these can cause brain and nerve damage. Marijuana, for example, so favored by college students who are supposed to be getting bright today so they can be the executives of tomorrow, has been reported capable of causing brain atrophy. Even schoolchildren have been shoved into drugs. And children of drug-taking mothers have been born as druggies.

I have even established that there is such a thing as a "drug personality." It is artificial and is created by drugs. Drugs can apparently change the attitude of a person from his original personality to one secretly harboring hostilities and hatreds he does not permit to show on the surface. While this may not hold true in all cases, it does establish a link between drugs and increasing difficulties with crime, production and the modern breakdown of social and industrial culture.

The devastating physiological effects of drugs are the subject of newspaper headlines routinely. That they also result in a breakdown of mental alertness and ethical fiber is all too obvious.

The drug scene is planetwide. It is swimming in blood and human misery.

But, vicious and damaging though they are, street drugs are actually only one part of the biochemical problem.

MEDICAL AND PSYCHIATRIC DRUGS

Medical and most particularly psychiatric drugs (Valium, Librium and LSD to name but a few) can be every bit as damaging as street drugs. The prevalence of these currently in common use would be quite amazing to one unfamiliar with the problem.

Phenobarbital[1] (under various brand names like Luminal and Nembutal) and other such drugs are often administered as though they were a panacea for all ills. As early as 1951 many persons had become so accustomed to their daily dosage of sleeping pills or painkillers that they did not consider their little pills as drugs. More recently the drug Valium has taken its place among the tranquilizers[2] so frequently employed. But this by no means completes the list.

Too often the attitude is "If I can't find the cause of the pain, at least I'll deaden it." In the case of one mentally ill, this might read, "If he can't be made rational, at least he can be made quiet."

1. **phenobarbital:** a white crystalline powder used as a sedative and hypnotic.
2. **tranquilizers:** drugs that have a sedative or calming effect without inducing sleep.

Unfortunately, it is not recognized that a person whose pain has been deadened by a sedative has himself been deadened by the same drug, and is much nearer the ultimate pain of death. It should be obvious that the quietest people in the world are the dead.

COMMERCIAL PROCESSES AND PRODUCTS

In recent years much research has been done on the potential toxic effects of many of the substances commonly used in various commercial processes and products, and to what extent they may be finding their way into the bodies of this planet's inhabitants. Following are a few examples of what this research has brought to light.

Industrial Chemicals: Under this heading exists a vast array of chemicals that are used in manufacturing. Not all such chemicals are toxic, of course. But workers in factories which produce or use such things as pesticides, petroleum products, plastics, detergents and cleaning chemicals, solvents, plated metals, preservatives, drugs, asbestos products, fertilizers, some cosmetics, perfumes, paints, dyes, electrical equipment or any radioactive materials can be exposed, often for extended periods, to toxic materials. And of course, the consumer can be exposed to residual amounts of such chemicals when he uses these products.

Agricultural Chemicals: Pesticides are the most obvious of the toxic substances to which workers in agricultural activities could be exposed. These include insecticides (insect-killing chemicals), man-made fertilizers and herbicides (chemicals to kill unwanted plants such as weeds).

Under the heading of herbicides come several which contain a substance known as "dioxin," known to be a highly toxic chemical, even in amounts almost too small to detect in the body. (Dioxin is found in "Agent Orange," a chemical defoliant used in the Vietnam

War. This chemical was the subject of considerable publicity when it was found that some US soldiers were exposed to it, apparently with varying adverse effects.)

Contact with chemicals used in agriculture can occur in a number of ways: The chemical can be carried on or in the plant itself and so eaten; it can be carried on the wind and be breathed in directly by those living or working in agricultural areas; or it can even be carried into drinking water supplies.

Food, Food Additives and Preservatives: There are substances added to some commercially processed foods that are meant to "enhance" color or flavor or, as mentioned above, to keep the food from spoiling. Also becoming more common are various artificial sweeteners used in "diet" soft drinks and other commercially packaged foods. From research on these "enhancers" and "preservers," it appears that a number of them are quite toxic, and the whole subject of food additives and preservatives has become a matter of concern to many people.

There is another side to this matter of food. Research findings point to the possibility that rancid oils are a health hazard of a magnitude not previously suspected. Oils used in cooking or commercial processing of foods, where they are not fresh, pure and free of rancidity, have been linked by researchers with digestive and muscular ills, and even cancer.

Perfumes and Fragrances: Use of perfumes and fragrances in all sorts of products has become more and more prevalent in recent years. Everything from clothing to laundry detergent, from cellophane tape to wrapping paper is turning up with *fragrance* added to it. And that fragrance is almost always a cheap chemical derivative, an extract of coal tar which probably costs about 10 cents a fifty-gallon drum. Findings seem to bear out that these chemicals, floating about in the local supermarket as "fragrances," are actually toxic *and* can end up in the food products sold there.

And when you get a mouthful of this stuff it is no aid to digestion, believe me!

Radiation: You've no doubt seen in news publications that contact with radiation can occur through exposure to nuclear weapons tests or the radioactive particles they can release into the atmosphere, nuclear wastes, or to some manufacturing processes which use radioactive materials. There are other sources of radiation exposure, too: prolonged exposure to the sun, dental and medical X-rays, television sets and unshielded computer display screens are among them.

Recent research has been done into a naturally occurring radioactive gas known as radon. It is a product of the decay of another radioactive element, radium, which has been found to be present in minute amounts in the ground and in many building materials such as concrete, brick and gravel. Apparently, tiny amounts of radon gas can escape from the surfaces of such materials and thus be present in the air and inhaled. If ventilation is not provided for, the radon content of the air in a building can reportedly reach 50 to 100 times the level found outdoors.

These factors are *all* part of the biochemical problem.

Any of these substances reportedly has the potential of remaining in the system.

This compounds the biochemical problem and presents a barrier of magnitude.

The most likely place for a toxic substance to lock up is in the fatty tissue. It has been said that in middle age and past middle age, a body's ability to break down fat lessens. So here we have, apparently, a situation of toxic substances locked up in fatty tissue and the fatty tissue is not actually getting broken down, and so such toxic substances could accumulate.

My interest in these somewhat brutal truths was not born only of an objective to resolve the physical ills of individuals. Rather, it was a continuation of my initial research involving the freeing of man as a spirit and handling, on this route, any barriers needing to be resolved.

The Purification program is a proffered answer to the barrier we call the biochemical problem. It could be called a "long-range detoxification program." While it is addressed primarily to the handling of drug residues lodged in the body, it is possible that there are many toxic substances which the body accumulates which the program may accelerate getting rid of.

My concern in developing the Purification program has not been with handling bodies. My research for many, many years has been carried out with the purpose of freeing man spiritually. My original inquiry was into the nature of man and the bulk of my work has always addressed man as a spiritual being. When barriers to this have arisen, those barriers have merited further research and resolution.

The Purification program was developed to meet a growing threat to mental and spiritual advancement and well-being stemming from the more and more common use of drugs and biochemical substances in the current culture.

Its procedures do not supplant technology developed earlier, used especially in Narconon[3] drug rehabilitation centers for handling persons currently on drugs and apt to experience withdrawal symptoms when taken off them. The Purification program would be begun only after such technology was applied.

---

3. **Narconon:** a social betterment organization and global network of drug rehabilitation and drug education centers, dedicated to restoring drug-free lives to drug dependent people through the use of L. Ron Hubbard's drug rehabilitation methods.

There are no medicines or drugs used on the Purification program. The only dosages recommended are those classified as food. There are no medical recommendations or claims made for the program. The only claim is future spiritual improvement.

The data contained herein is a record of researches and results noted; it cannot be construed as a recommendation for medical treatment or medication, and it is undertaken or delivered by any individual on his own responsibility.

If the Purification program can be used to salvage even a part of a civilization sick from the onslaught of drugs and other toxic substances, then perhaps there is hope for all of that civilization.

∽

CHAPTER TWO

THE DEVELOPMENT OF THE PURIFICATION PROGRAM

WHAT IS THE PURIFICATION PROGRAM?

To state it simply, it is a program developed to assist in releasing and flushing out of the body the accumulated toxic residues which may be lodged in the tissues, while also rebuilding the impaired tissues and cells.

What is its genesis?

DISCOVERY THAT LSD CAN LODGE IN THE SYSTEM

In the 1970s, working with cases of individuals who had been drug users, and in a study of their physical symptoms and behavioral patterns, I made a startling discovery.

People who had been on LSD at some earlier time sometimes had reactions which appeared to act as if they had just taken more LSD!

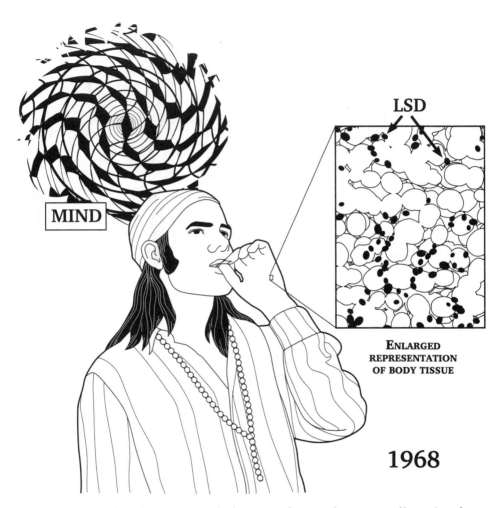

LSD

MIND

ENLARGED
REPRESENTATION
OF BODY TISSUE

1968

As it has been stated that it takes only one millionth of an ounce of LSD to produce a drugged condition and because it is basically wheat rust,[1] which simply cuts off circulation, my original thinking on this was that LSD must remain in the body.

1. **wheat rust:** a fungus which attacks wheat and produces reddish, brown or black marks resembling iron rust on the stems and leaves. The fungus penetrates the plant and forms a mass of filaments (the threadlike parts of a fungus) within the invaded tissue, and thus absorbs nourishment.

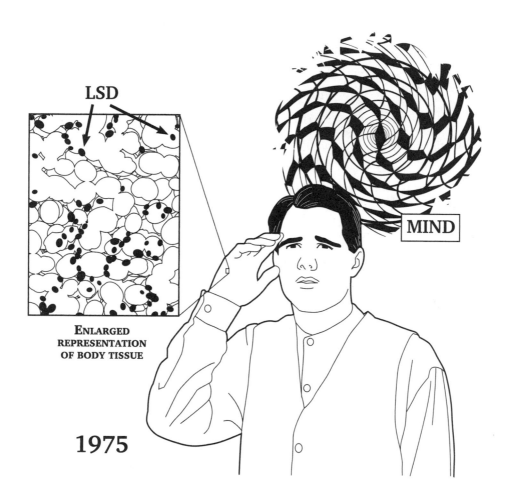

LSD

ENLARGED
REPRESENTATION
OF BODY TISSUE

MIND

1975

In other words:

LSD apparently stays in the system, lodging in the tissues, and mainly the fatty tissues of the body, and is liable to go into action again—giving the person unpredictable "trips"—even years after the person has come off LSD.

This was an observable phenomenon—dramatically so!

In the face of this discovery, was it then also possible that residues of other drugs could lock up in the system and at some point reactivate with similar, if less dramatic, effect?

And if so, how did one then ever fully free people from the effects of drugs? Were they simply doomed thereafter to be at the effect of drugs whenever these residues chanced to reactivate?

What of the other debilitating effects of the presence of these drug residues? It was known that drugs burn up vitamin reserves. What other physical consequences might stem from the hidden presence of such drug deposits?

One could not ignore the possibility that, even when "dormant"—if that expression can indeed ever be used for a toxic substance—they might be highly damaging to the organism.

And what of the potential spiritual and mental growth of individuals so affected? For it was also an observable fact that one was faced with some unchanging characteristics in a certain number of these cases, even when much of the mental and spiritual trauma of drug experiences had apparently been relieved. Among these characteristics was a "woodenness" of personality and a noticeable difficulty in the ability to absorb and comprehend or retain and apply new data—in other words, an impaired ability to learn or change.

What was the answer to these cases?

No known method existed for ridding the body of these minute drug deposits which, locked as they were in the tissues, were not totally dispelled in the normal processes of elimination.

The answer obviously did not lie in attempting to handle with more drugs or biochemicals which would only compound the situation.

But could a method be evolved to dislodge and flush them out, thereby freeing the person for full rehabilitation physically as well as mentally and spiritually?

The Original "Sweat Program"

Operating on the premise that the negative factors observed might be reversed if there were a means of getting LSD deposits out of the system, and that the most logical method to accomplish this would be to sweat them out, I worked out and released in 1977 a regimen called "The Sweat Program." Utilized mainly by those who had been heavily into drugs, particularly LSD, the procedure produced positive results. With it, evidences of the release of residues of other types of street drugs began to appear.

The regimen was a lengthy process, however, taking months to complete. A refinement and speedup was needed.

Discovery of Other Embedded Toxins

Using data and proven theories from earlier researches over the years, development was begun of a more comprehensive program, broader nutritionally and more streamlined.

From its earliest application another factor emerged which tended to support the theories upon which this new program was based: persons on the research program were reporting the apparent exudation[2] of substances other than just street drugs—substances smelling or tasting or feeling like medicines, anesthetics, diet pills, food preservatives, pesticides and any number of other chemical preparations in common use!

The list included not only LSD, heroin, cocaine, marijuana and "angel dust," but many other biochemical substances—medicinal and pharmaceutical drugs such as aspirin and codeine, as well as commercial and agricultural and industrial chemicals.

These same persons were also experiencing, in mild form, some of the sensations of old sunburns, past illnesses and injuries and other past conditions, both physical and emotional.

Thus it seems that residues of any or all of these hostile biochemical substances apparently have the potential of remaining in the system, getting caught up in the tissues and remaining there, unsuspected, even after they have supposedly been eliminated from the body years earlier.

Their accumulation, unhandled, probably disarranges the biochemistry and fluid balance of the body.

This was my early thinking on the subject. It was now being borne out by further research, as more and more manifestations occurred. (It has also since been borne out by clinical tests and by medical autopsies which have found deposits of certain drugs embedded in body tissues.)

---

2. **exudation:** the action of coming out gradually in drops, as sweat, through pores or small openings; oozing out.

With the ongoing research, all indicators were that these substances were being flushed out as people progressed on the program. And these same individuals were reporting that they felt a new vigor, a renewed vitality and interest in life.

With a large number of people coming successfully through the regimen the research was completed.

The Purification program was released.

ELEMENTS OF THE PURIFICATION PROGRAM

The Purification program is a precisely designed regimen. It includes the following elements:

• Exercise, in the form of running, to stimulate the circulation.

• Prescribed periods in a sauna, which, accompanied by certain vitamins and other nutrients, enable one to sweat out the accumulated toxins.

• A nutritional program, including:

One's regular diet which is then supplemented with plenty of fresh vegetables which are not overcooked.

An exact regimen of vitamin, mineral and oil intake.

Sufficient liquids to offset the loss of body fluids through sweating.

A properly ordered personal schedule which provides the person with the normally required amount of sleep.

These are not unfamiliar actions to the majority of us.

How then can they accomplish what they apparently do? Why this particular set of actions? How is it that these elements, combined, might accomplish what no one of them apparently, singly or even in other combinations, has accomplished heretofore?

While the procedures to be followed are not unusual, the answers to these questions lie in the very exact combination of the elements which make up the program, in the properties of the nutrients used in specific increments and in the increased proportions of these in exact ratio to each other, as laid out in detail in the next chapters of this book.

WARNING

There is a warning which should be stressed in any description of this program. That is, simple and familiar as the outlined actions may appear:

They must be followed exactly for the best possible results.

Because of the technical nature of the program, and because it is a strenuous program it must only be undertaken after a physical examination and written approval from an advised medical doctor.

Anyone with a weak heart or who is anemic or who suffers from certain kidney conditions, for example, should not do this program but would require a similar but special program of a milder nature.

Additionally, while doing the program people have reported *reexperiencing* various effects of past drugs, medicine, alcohol or other stimulants or sedatives—including full-blown drug "trips." For this reason, and for its success on any individual, it is best done under the close supervision of persons trained and experienced in its administration.

Also, even with this tight supervision, one does not do the actions by himself but always carries these out accompanied by a partner.

᠙

CHAPTER THREE

HOW THE PURIFICATION PROGRAM WORKS

HOW DOES THE PURIFICATION PROGRAM WORK?

Running is done to get the blood circulating deeper into the tissues where toxic residuals are lodged and thus act to loosen and release the accumulated harmful deposits and get them moving.

Very important, then, is that the running is immediately followed by sweating in the sauna to flush out the accumulations which have now been dislodged.

Regular nutrition and supplemental nutrition in the form of megavitamin and mineral dosages and extra quantities of oil are a vital factor in helping the body to flush out toxins and to repair and rebuild the areas that have been affected by drugs and other toxic residuals.

A proper schedule with enough rest is mandatory, as the body will be undergoing change and repair throughout the program.

These actions, carried out on a very stringently monitored basis, are apparently accomplishing a detoxification of the entire system, to the renewed mental and physical vigor of the individual.

There is a more in-depth view to be taken of the entire process, however.

A person who has taken drugs, in addition to the physical factors involved, retains *mental image pictures* of those drugs and their effects. Mental image pictures are three-dimensional color pictures with sound and smell and all other perceptions, plus the conclusions or speculations of the individual. They are mental copies of one's perceptions sometime in the past. For example, a person who had taken LSD would retain "pictures" of that experience in his mind, complete with recordings of the sights, physical sensations, smells, sounds, etc., that occurred while he was under the influence of LSD.

Let us say an individual took LSD one day while at a fairground with some friends, and the day's experiences included feeling nauseated and dizzy, getting into an argument with a friend, feeling an emotion of sadness, and later feeling very tired. He would have mental image pictures of that entire incident.

Such mental image pictures can be reactivated by drug residuals, as the presence of these drugs in the tissues of the body can simulate the earlier drug experiences. This is known as *restimulation:* the reactivation of a past memory due to similar circumstances in the present approximating circumstances of the past.

Using the above example of the person who took LSD, sometime later—perhaps years afterward—the residuals of the drug that are still in his body tissues can cause a restimulation of that LSD incident. The mental image pictures are reactivated, and he experiences the same sensations of nausea, dizziness and tiredness, and he feels sad. He does not know why. He might also perceive mental images of the persons he was with and the accompanying sights and sounds and smells.

Therefore, on the Purification program we are looking at two things: one, the actual drugs and toxic residuals in the body (and medical autopsies have shown that they are there); and two, the mental image pictures of the drugs and the mental image pictures of one's experiences with these drugs.

These two factors are hung up, one playing against the other, in perfect balance. What the person is feeling is the two conditions, one of them the actual presence of the drug residuals, the other the mental image pictures relating to them.

Probably the reason why the Purification program works is that it handles the one side of it—the accumulated toxic residuals—and thus fixes the person up so that the other side, the mental image picture side of it, is no longer in constant restimulation. It is as simple as that.

What, among other things, is happening on the Purification program is that you cause an upset of this perfect balance. Suddenly the balance isn't there anymore so you don't get the cross reaction anymore. The harmful and restimulative chemical residues have been flushed out—they're gone. This does not mean the mental image pictures are gone. But they are no longer in restimulation and they're not being reinforced by the presence of drug residuals.

By breaking up the balance of these two and handling the one side of it on the Purification program we are freeing the person up for mental and spiritual gain.

MENTAL IMAGE PICTURES

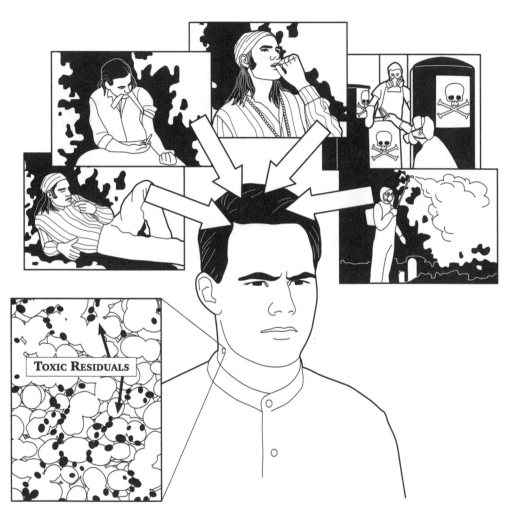

TOXIC RESIDUALS

ENLARGED
REPRESENTATION
OF BODY TISSUE

"Therefore, on the Purification program we are looking at two things: one, the actual drugs and toxic residuals in the body (and medical autopsies have shown that they are there); and two, the mental image pictures of the drugs and the mental image pictures of one's experiences with these drugs."

26

MENTAL IMAGE PICTURES

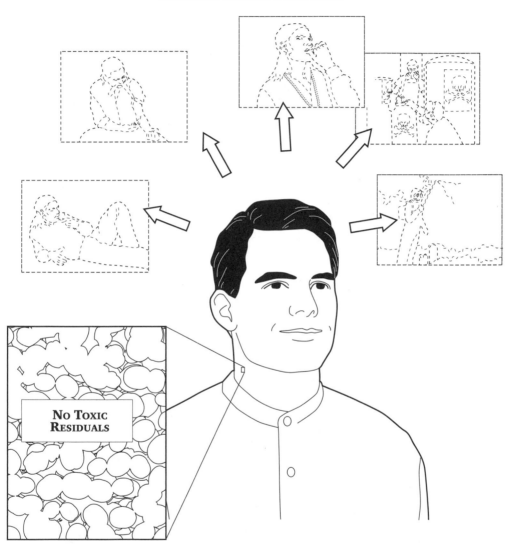

ENLARGED
REPRESENTATION
OF BODY TISSUE

"Probably the reason why the Purification program works is that it handles the one side of it—the accumulated toxic residuals—and thus fixes the person up so that the other side, the mental image picture side of it, is no longer in constant restimulation. It is as simple as that."

A "LONG-RANGE DETOXIFICATION" PROGRAM

Drug residues can stop any mental or spiritual help. They also stop a person's life! While originally addressed primarily to the handling of the accumulation of drugs in the system, it appears from the research results recorded and noted above that with use of this regimen many other toxic substances accumulated by the body can be flushed out of the system.

These substances must be eliminated if one is to get stable mental and spiritual improvement. The operating rule is that mental actions and even biophysical actions—methods of bringing an individual into better communication with his environment—do not work in the presence of life-hostile elements.

In rehabilitating an individual, only when we have accomplished a biochemical handling can we then go on to the next step, the biophysical handling (improving the person's ability to handle his body and environment) and then on to mental and spiritual improvement.

When one tries to move these around and put them out of sequence, one gets losses.

The development of a program to handle drugs and drug and chemical deposits in the body was based on the fact that successful rehabilitation of an individual can only be accomplished in the sequence outlined above.

Apparent gain occurs by cleaning up the body and can be seen as an end-all in itself, though that was not the original motivation.

In view of what it evidently accomplishes, the Purification program might be termed a long-range detoxification program.

But it should be identified as itself, since it is unique among detoxification programs, both in its procedure and reported results. To my knowledge, there is no other known method by which these locked-in accumulations may be gotten out of the body.

CHAPTER FOUR

FLUSHING OUT TOXINS

O N THE PURIFICATION PROGRAM, in order to flush the drugs and other toxins out of the body, a combination of *exercise,* in the form of running, and *sauna* is essential. These are done for a five-hour period daily, in a ratio of approximately:

> *twenty to thirty minutes of running, to*
> *four to four and one-half hours sauna time.*

The ratio is emphasized here as the bulk of the period is best spent in the sauna after the circulation has been worked up by running. In other words, the five-hour period is *not* 50 percent exercising and 50 percent sauna. The program gives best results with a much lower percentage of time exercising and a much higher percentage in the sauna.

SAFEGUARD: WORKING WITH A PARTNER

Running and sauna sweat-out should *always* be done with another person, as restimulation of past drugs, medicines, alcohol or even anesthetics can and does occur as the toxins get flushed out. This can include the restimulation of a full-blown "trip" from LSD or other drugs one may have taken.

Pairing up on the program so that one is *always* doing the running and sauna steps with a partner or even a third person, provides a safety factor in the case of any of the above eventualities.

RUNNING

The first action on the program itself is running. The purpose of this is *not* to generate sweat but to get the blood circulating and the system functioning so that impurities held in the system can be released and pumped out.

Running increases the circulation throughout the whole body, thus:

a. it causes cell waste to be carried out more rapidly, and

b. it causes the circulation to go deeper into the muscles and tissues so that those areas which have been stagnant can now get rid of the accumulation of biochemical deposits and, in the case of LSD, the "residual crystals" which have been stored.

Running is done on a daily basis once the person has begun the program.

The running should be done on a gradient. If one is so breathless that he can't talk to another while running then he is straining too much, so the running should be taken on a lower gradient.

SWEATING IN THE SAUNA

The second action, which directly follows the running, is sweating. A person goes into the sauna immediately after running in order to sweat. The impurities which have been freed up by the increased circulation can now be dispelled from the system and leave the body through the pores.

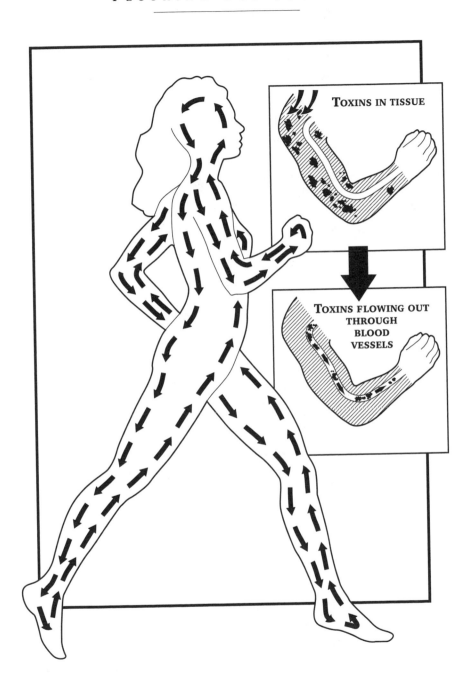

TOXINS IN TISSUE

TOXINS FLOWING OUT
THROUGH
BLOOD
VESSELS

Sweating in the sauna is done at temperatures ranging anywhere from 140 degrees to 180 degrees. It is a matter of what temperature the person can take. Usually, but not always, a person beginning the program will start at a lower temperature and work up to a higher temperature. Then as he progresses he will find he can take increasing degrees of heat.

CLOTHING

Running is usually done in a regular sweat suit. This is optional, however, depending upon the geographical location, season or weather.

In the sauna one would simply wear a swimming suit or swimming trunks or some similar light apparel.

And, while it may seem almost absurd to include the following datum here, it has been included as the mistake was made (and swiftly corrected) in one area shortly following the initial release of the Purification program:

A sweat suit is *never* worn in the sauna. The reason for this is that a sweat suit acts as insulation, much the same as when a diver wears a wet suit for insulation against the cold of the sea. Wearing a sweat suit would insulate one against the heat of the sauna and so inhibit and curtail sweating.

LIQUIDS

While on this program, it is important that one drink plenty of water, which greatly assists in flushing and cleansing the system. Additionally, with all the sweating done in the sauna it would be dangerous not to replenish body fluids. So a good amount of water, and any other nonalcoholic liquids the person might choose, should be taken daily.

RADIATION AND LIQUIDS

On the Purification program, findings seem to bear out that there is a factor related to radiation that produces the greatest exudation of it and that is the sweating itself.

Radiation is apparently enormously water-soluble as well as water removable. According to researchers, one merely has to take a hose to a building surface or a road to wash the radiation off of it. This factor is well known to defense trained personnel.

So where one is doing the Purification program, one should be very careful to ensure that actual sweating occurs and in volume. A sufficient intake of water is therefore quite vital when doing the program.

This has a side effect, however, of washing a lot of minerals out of the system and perhaps vitamins, as well. Thus the intake of minerals and vitamins during the program is also a necessity.

It is possible that the Purification program is not as workable when profuse sweating does not occur, when liquid intake is not large enough to compensate for it and when vitamins and minerals of a water-soluble nature are not carefully and adequately replaced. (The common vitamins taken on the Purification program which are not water-soluble are vitamins A, D and E.)

This gives us three important points which must be in on a Purification program:

1. Profuse sweating must occur.

2. A person's liquid intake must be large enough to compensate for the liquid lost through sweating.

3. Vitamins and minerals must be taken in sufficient quantities to replace those washed out of the system through sweating.

As megavitamin dosages are also a part of the Purification program, this mineral and vitamin intake is quite in addition to any other vitamin therapy ongoing at the time.

OVERHEATING

One could get overheated in the sauna if it is not taken on the right gradient.

When a person gets too warm or begins feeling faint, should the body temperature get too high, the recommendation is to go out and take a cool shower and then go back into the sauna. People who are having a hard time spending consecutive hours in the sauna will be able to handle the sauna time if a cooling shower is taken when needed.

SALT OR POTASSIUM DEPLETION

Extra salt (sodium chloride) is not mandatory for every individual on the program. But salt and potassium are lost in sweating. Thus, one must watch for any symptoms of salt or potassium depletion and remedy the depletion at once, should it occur.

The symptoms can be similar to those of overheating or, when extreme, similar to the symptoms of heat exhaustion (clammy skin, extreme tiredness, weakness, headache and sometimes cramps, nausea, dizziness, vomiting or even fainting).

Such manifestations would be handled immediately with extra salt or salt tablets, potassium gluconate tablets, Bioplasma,[1] or "salt substitute" which is mainly potassium.

A supply of these substances must be readily available at all times to anyone who is doing the Purification program. Ideally,

---

1. **Bioplasma:** a trademark name of a dietary supplement containing a combination of mineral salts, which the body uses.

supplies of these would be located right outside the sauna, clearly labeled as to what they are.

It is a matter of good common sense that overheating and salt or potassium depletion can be *prevented* by sufficient salt, potassium or Bioplasma taken periodically while in the sauna and by cooling off when it becomes necessary during the sauna time. But should these symptoms occur, they must be handled and not considered something the person must "go through."

Also, one must guard against falling asleep in the sauna, as overheating or salt or potassium depletion could occur while one was asleep.

Salt or potassium depletion as a *chronic condition* must be handled as a separate factor by a medical doctor.

HEATSTROKE

If perspiration ceases while in the sauna—the body suddenly stops sweating and the skin becomes hot and dry—it's an indicator that needs immediate handling. This is a clamping down on the part of the body, a resistance to expelling, and it is the first sign of heatstroke.

The *Standard First Aid Personal Safety Booklet* put out by the American National Red Cross covers the symptoms of heat exhaustion and/or heatstroke and the immediate aid to be given for such.

One would get the person out of the sauna at once and cool him off with a lukewarm or cool shower or sponging, or start with a lukewarm shower and gradually make it cooler. Fluids and salt, potassium or Bioplasma would be given.

The first aid safety booklet must be kept on hand as a reference, readily available, in the sauna location.

DRY SAUNA VERSUS WET SAUNA

Thus far, the use of a dry sauna has proved to be the most successful in inducing profuse sweating in most people. It is possible that some may sweat more in a wet sauna; it has not yet been fully tested. It may be that it is an individual matter. There is no regulation on the program that outlaws the use of a wet sauna. Whichever type of sauna is employed, the whole idea is to use the system which permits the person to sweat the most.

Steam baths, at similar temperatures to the sauna, can be used by themselves when available. They serve much the same purpose as the dry sauna and it has been suggested that a steam bath may even work faster, but this has not been confirmed. The steam bath produces a similar effect. Thus, either can be used.

The same precautions apply to the use of a steam bath as to the sauna.

EUCALYPTUS OIL

A small quantity of eucalyptus oil is sometimes added to the steam in a steam bath or similarly used in some saunas.

In a modern sauna or steam bath, the procedure is to simply put one or two capfuls of eucalyptus oil in a bucket of water in the room. As it then evaporates (the oil will evaporate before the water does), more can be added as needed.

Some people don't like the smell of eucalyptus at all, while others find it pleasant. If the solution is too strong it can cause watering of the eyes or nausea in some cases. Thus, one would survey before using it and, if used, it should be in appropriate small quantities.

Used correctly, eucalyptus has been reported to be beneficial in clearing up the lungs and clearing the sinuses. One person has reported his voice smoothing out as a result of using eucalyptus oil in the sauna.

It is not a mandatory step on the Purification program, but the data given here on the use of eucalyptus oil in the sauna or steam bath, as an optional element, should be known.

Whether or not eucalyptus is used, it goes without saying that a sauna or steam bath should be kept hygienic and free of odors by having the room scrubbed at least once, or oftener, daily.

∾

CHAPTER FIVE

IMPORTANCE OF A PROPER SCHEDULE

THE PROPERLY ORDERED PERSONAL SCHEDULE required while one is on the Purification program consists of:

a. a sufficient amount of sleep daily.

b. correct ratio of running time to sauna time, and the total prescribed period for these adhered to daily.

c. sticking to the program sensibly and not skipping days or skimping or shortcutting on the prescribed daily schedule, nor doing any part of the program in a random fashion.

Ideally, this includes getting in the exercise (running) and sauna time at approximately the same time each day; and taking the vitamin and mineral nutrients at approximately the same time each day, as when these factors are kept in predictably the program goes much more smoothly.

SLEEP

The need for adequate sleep should be emphasized here as it has been found to be a vital, vital factor in the application of the program. People function best when they are sufficiently rested.

Eight hours of sleep is considered the usual daily requirement. Some persons may need more than this, but getting less than the regular amount of sleep one usually requires is not advised.

Some tiredness has not been uncommon at certain intervals during the course of the program even when the procedure was being carried out totally standardly. It can occur when the individual first goes onto the program and is not up to doing a five-hour stint per day, in which case the person should build up to the full daily period on a gradient by doing a bit more time each successive day until he is able to do the full five hours. It can also occur as part of the restimulation in connection with medical or street drug residues or as part of the restimulation of an old illness, etc., any of which the person might run through while on this program. There are cases on record of persons going through periods of tiredness or fatigue connected with past illness and/or medical or drug experiences and coming through them far brighter and more energetic.

But it must be borne in mind that the Purification program can be strenuous. Trying to do it on too little sleep would be a severe violation of the regulations covering the program. A person obviously needs enough sleep and rest in order to cope with the changes taking place in his body and in order to assist the body in any needed rebuild of tissues or cellular repair. Per Program Case Supervisor[1] reports, where a schedule for sufficient sleep has been violated the person has often wound up having a rough time of it, which is totally unnecessary. Quite apart from any mere tiredness, any reactions which are there to be restimulated by drug residues can, due to insufficient sleep and rest, produce unnecessary and nonoptimum reactions.

One obviously cannot expect to make the gains that are possible on the Purification program unless this point is in.

---

1. **Program Case Supervisor:** a properly certified person who is assigned the responsibility of overseeing the delivery of and ensuring the proper and exact application of all aspects of the Purification program to individuals.

OPTIMUM DAILY TIME ON THE PROGRAM

From the many cases interviewed and from data from those who have supervised the program, five hours exercise and sauna daily has been found to be ideal for the majority of people doing the Purification program. The program apparently works like a bomb[2] when the highest percentage of this time is spent in the sauna and a lesser percentage in running. (Example: A good ratio has been found to be approximately 20 to 30 minutes of running to get the circulation up, followed by the remainder of the time spent in the sauna, for a total of five hours.)

Not everyone has gone immediately onto a full five-hour stint right from the start. (And some have successfully done the program on a shorter daily schedule.)

In both the running and the sauna, where the right gradient was applied—particularly when beginning the program—it went very smoothly.

AGE AND PHYSICAL CONDITION—
FACTORS IN SCHEDULING

Age, physical condition and stamina can all enter into it, and these factors would need to be taken into consideration for each program participant individually when starting the person on the program.

Among the many people surveyed on program results were those who had required a few days to work up to five hours daily. However, once up to the five-hour daily schedule, that proved to be the optimum daily period for those persons, as it has for so many of the people who have been through the program.

Additionally, on such a schedule the Purification program can and has been completed effectively in the shortest possible amount of time.

---

2. **like a bomb:** with considerable effectiveness or overwhelming success.

Most people approached the five-hour daily program eagerly and enthusiastically.

Some eager beavers were found apt to plunge in a bit too quickly at the start, and this was handled by having them work up gradually to where they could run 20 to 30 minutes without strain while at the same time increasing the sauna time gradually up to the full prescribed period.

One Program Case Supervisor reported a few people staying in the sauna too long with no break and turning on headaches and other unnecessary reactions as a result. The purpose should not be to see how long one can stay in the sauna for any one stretch of time—and this had to be clarified with several such enthusiasts.

What worked best was when the person had been in the sauna sweating for a while and had a good sweat going and then came out, got some fresh air and space and cooled off, as needed. Then he or she went right back into the sauna for more sweating. When plenty of liquids (many people take water jugs into the sauna with them) and enough salt, potassium and Bioplasma were used, the sauna time went very well.

HOW LONG DOES THE PURIFICATION PROGRAM TAKE?

With each of the points of the program kept in and the regimen followed exactly, the program can be completed by many at five hours a day in two or three weeks' time.

Some persons may take a bit more time than that; a few might complete the program in less time.

CHAPTER SIX

NUTRITION

Nutrition plays a vital role in the Purification program. But when we speak of nutrition in relation to the program we are not talking only about food in the most common usage of the word. We are talking about vitamins and minerals as well.

Regular Eating Habits

There are *no* "special diets" required on this program.

The person simply eats what he normally would, supplemented with plenty of vegetables which have not been overcooked and with the recommended dosages of vitamins and minerals.

There is no thought here of putting the person on any kind of special diet at all. There are no restrictions on what one may eat. We are not even trying to preach against toxic foods or campaign against diet abuses or junk foods or anything of that sort.

We are only trying to handle the *accumulation* of impurities built up in the body. If one wanted to defend his body against all future impurities then that is another program and not part of this one.

To put a person on a diet different than that to which he is accustomed is to introduce a sudden change in the midst of other changes he will be experiencing on the program. A change of diet might be just one too many changes and would be an additive[1] which could interfere with and affect the efficacy of the program.

DIETS AND FOOD FADS

I am not a food faddist and there is no idea of mixing any food fad into this program. However, there is plenty of food faddism going on in society and you can easily start such a fad, so this must be watched when administering the Purification program. There is no intention to have people eating banana fronds split into diamonds and star shapes and blessed by some deity or other, or a fad of "three lettuce leaves crisscrossed with two slabs of peanut butter as an absolute must eighteen times a day," or something equally silly being touted as "the only food a person can have."

Food is subject to becoming very faddist and, frankly, most people know very little about it.

Locating and remedying deficiencies and excesses in vitamins, minerals, enzymes, sugar, protein, oil and fats, carbohydrates and bulk fiber[2] as well as other dietary supplements is the keynote of dieting. No special substance or food or abstinence from it is a whole answer.

Diets should be considered a subject where one seeks a balance of body support elements and determines quantity.

Fasting, magic foods eaten to the exclusion of others and dozens of dietary fads alike tend to be more harmful than beneficial.

1. **additive:** a thing which has been added. This usually has a bad meaning in that an additive is said to be something needless or harmful which has been done in addition to standard procedure. Additive normally means a departure from standard procedure.
2. **bulk fiber:** the structural part of plants and plant products that are wholly or partially indigestible and when eaten help to move waste products through the intestines; roughage.

There is a vast difference between food-faddism and the subject of diets. Diets have become viewed as what a person is *limited to* in eating, whereas they should be viewed as what a person *must have* as nutritional elements. This has become a problem because the true natural diet of man has not been isolated.

THEORY OF A NATURAL DIET

Food, lack of it, incorrect planning or consumption of it or substitution or alteration of it can vastly affect health.

Man is not a primary converter of natural energy or masses but depends upon other converters for a primary conversion in most cases. (Except for vitamin D and one or two other items man, for instance, does not convert sunlight to energy, but, eating algae which does so convert, is able to obtain and use the energy.)

No real study of or search for the natural diet of man has ever been made or attempted. Studies are made of diets from the viewpoint of how to correct illnesses or maintain health but not what the basic food of the human body would be. Scarcities, availabilities, what can be grown and preserved, the ease of growing, climatic and soil and water conditions, and how to make a profit are factors which have established diet instead of "What does the human body require?"

The human body is a complex biological carbon-oxygen engine, one running at an operating temperature of 37 degrees centigrade and, being biological, has the ability to establish and repair itself. To its food requirements then are added the elements required to build as well as to run the body.

Almost all mammals live about six times their period of growth. Man lives only three and one-third times his growth period. As other mammals than man are under the same or greater stress, but are usually uniform in diet while healthy, it can be assumed that man has departed from his natural diet.

Some guesses have been made as to natural diet by an examination of teeth but this would not be an adequate approach.

The resolution of man's natural diet as opposed to what he is eating might do a very great deal to improving racial health.

Man's mass efforts towards diet are targeted for quantity and profit. Efforts to establish quality are often resisted by various special interests in the mistaken idea that further knowledge of diet might reduce quantity and profit. However, it could be that new food discoveries would vastly increase both production quantity potential and profit.

No simple basis for research and discovery of the natural diet exists in known statement form. The necessary first steps to the discovery of man's correct diet would be:

a. The statement of a possibility that one might have existed or did exist.

b. A formula for search and possible discovery of it.

This section of the book has made (a) above.

The following would be a formula for its discovery:

Overweight: Residual elements of food, substances or gases which are not totally eliminated or utilized by the body after ingestion.

Underweight or debility: Inadequate or lacking foods, substances or gases which are needed for the activity, maintenance or repair of the body.

By listing all foods, substances or gases which are *stored* by the body, one would obtain a list of things ingested, part of which were not utilized or necessary. Simple recording of those items which put on unwanted weight would be a part of this action. The examination of overweight persons and their diets would give another section of it. Further examination of cadavers that had been overweight would round out the list. Which of these were the result of body conversion of what food would be noted.

A study and listing of all deficiency diseases and malnutrition cases as contained in *The Textbook of Medicine,* Beeson and McDermott, and in other papers and texts would give a list of items vital to the activity, maintenance and repair of the body.

The items in the overweight and debility lists could then be compared.

One would have, as a result, the elements of a natural diet.

A search for foods which contained *only* the elements which were *used* and *vital* could be undertaken.

The result would be the elements of a possible natural diet.

An examination of the ease of production and supply of such foods could then result in a practical natural diet.

Zonal application in specific areas might require the repetition of the formula to take in racial or climatic or production variables.

It is said that 80 percent of Americans are overweight. Their activity and intelligence are failing. The populations of many countries are starving or suffering malnutrition.

The wild animals, fish and fowl are ceasing to be a world source of food supply. There is no reason to go on killing off all life on the planet simply because no one knows, beyond opinion or taste, what man's natural food was or could be.

Fads and hobbies should not be the sole source of data on this subject.

The problem could be intelligently solved and should be if we are still to have a populated planet.

Probably the planet could support billions more than it does. Most of it is wasteland.

A system to solve it by killing off populations through sterilizing and euthanasia[3] is simply impractical, stupid and useless suppression.

It would be far better to work out man's natural diet.

This is quite another subject of research which could be undertaken by others whose primary field it is, but the discovery of such basics and making these widely known could result in a planetwide program which would at some future time decidedly augment the basic principles and implementation of the Purification program.

Meantime, it is not intended that dietary fads of any sort be included as part of the Purification program.

∽

___

3. **euthanasia:** the act or practice of painlessly putting to death an individual who is suffering from a terminal or incurable illness; "mercy killing." However, in the 1930s, a variation of euthanasia was used in Germany to rid the country of those considered burdens on society, including mentally defective people and alcoholics. Following on the heels of programs to sterilize people termed "unfit," euthanasia programs were employed in murdering over 200,000 mental patients from 1939 to 1945. These programs further expanded in the 1940s to include others considered "unworthy of life."

CHAPTER SEVEN

OIL: TRADING BAD FAT FOR GOOD FAT

TOXIC SUBSTANCES SEEM TO lock up mainly, but not exclusively, in the fat tissues of the body.

The theory is that one could replace the fat tissues that hold these accumulations with fat tissue which is free of such residues. It is a theory of exchange. It is based on the "Have–Waste" theory and formulas from my research in the 1950s, as described below.

HAVE–WASTE THEORY

Havingness is a term for a very fundamental principle which can be seen in operation in several different aspects of the Purification program.

Havingness has to do with a person's considerations in regard to mass. It means, to state it simply, the degree to which one is willing to experience mass—mass of any kind. One's degree of havingness is the degree that he is able to *have* or *not have* a particular thing, with no compulsion involved either way.

In good shape, a being should be able to experience anything. His recorded experience, however, may dictate otherwise.

His level of havingness is actually determined by his considerations on the subject. And his considerations can be influenced by a combination of factors, past and present. But the basic influencing factors in this are abundance and scarcity.

There is a little scale in operation here which was put to extensive test early in my work with people. While its application is broad, the simplicity of the scale, or formula, is just this:

Before a being can *have* something, he must be able to *waste* it.

If an individual can't *have* something, it is a cinch he'll *waste* it. And if he can't even waste it, it is a cinch he'll *substitute* for it.

We use this principle on the Purification program to effect the exchanges which are needed.

While the research and formulas of "Have–Waste" go very extensively into the subjects of being able to have, being able to waste and other aspects of these conditions, a very simple premise on which this theory can be explained is that:

Anything which is scarce becomes valuable.

The body will actually tend to hold on to something it is short of. Thus, if you try to get rid of something it is short of, it will resist giving it up.

The answer is to provide an additional supply of the substance.

Therefore, in the matter of fat, if the person takes some oil the body might possibly exchange the bad fat in the body for the good oil. That is the basic theory.

I am also indebted for material on this to a doctor in Portugal who, in conversation, told me that autopsies had found all sorts of grisly, used-up fat stored in unlikely places in people's bodies. In other words, there is a lot of unusable fat a body can accumulate.

The body will obviously hold on to a lot of fat and won't let go of it. The effort is to get the body to take good oil or fat in exchange for the bad, toxin-ridden fat it is holding on to. If one wants somebody to clean up the fat tissue in the body, he had better give

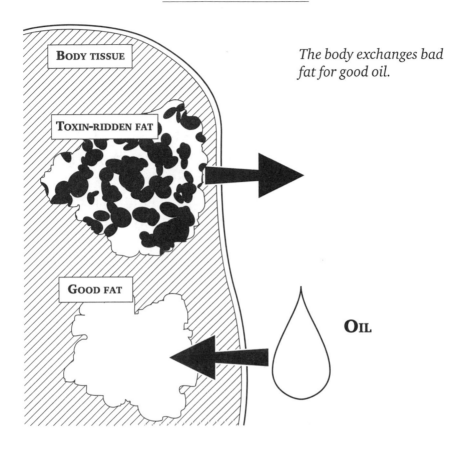

The body exchanges bad fat for good oil.

the body some fat in order to make up for the fat tissues the body is now, on the Purification program, releasing or changing.

In this way we have some chance of getting the body to release fatty tissue which is impregnated with toxic substances. We get the body to trade fat for fat.

OILS

One should use a blend of oils which contains soy, walnut, peanut and safflower oil.

Whether purchasing the oil in a health food or other type of store one should ensure it is fresh, not rancid.

If this type of oil is not obtainable in health food stores or elsewhere, one could blend it from these four oils in the proper amounts. Any oil used must be cold-pressed[1] and polyunsaturated,[2] and must be kept refrigerated so it remains fresh.

The oil used on the program must also include lecithin. Lecithin appears to be an agent capable of breaking fat into tiny particles which can pass readily into the tissues. It should be taken along with the oil on the Purification program, and is obtainable from most health food stores in a granulated form. The amount of lecithin to be taken has been estimated to be between one and two tablespoons per day, depending on how much oil one is taking. In its granulated form, it can be mixed with other food such as milk, yogurt or juice.

HOW MUCH OIL?

Upon initial release of the Purification program, the exact daily quantity of oil needed by a person on the program had not been definitely established, beyond the fact that it was very likely somewhere between two tablespoonfuls and one-half cup, depending upon the individual. One tablespoon of oil is not going to accomplish much, as too little oil won't let the body substitute good fat tissue for bad. If too much is given it can cause diarrhea.

A medical doctor who has handled numerous people on the program has reported that the most standard oil dosage found to be required by most persons he supervised on the program was between two and four tablespoonfuls a day. Others, particularly some 250-pounders under his care on the program, were on considerably more oil than that.

---

1. **cold-pressed:** produced through extraction by low pressure without generating much heat and as a result retaining its nutritional value.
2. **polyunsaturated:** designates types of fat or oil that chemically contain fewer hydrogen atoms than they could hold; *poly*—many, *unsaturated*—not filled to capacity. These oils are obtained primarily from vegetables. Some of them are fats and oils required by the body that must be supplied through the diet because the body is not able to manufacture them.

The recommendation of this medical doctor is that on an oil dosage of any quantity, one would reduce the oil intake if the oil showed up in a bowel movement or in the body sweat, as in such case there is an excess of oil which is not being put to use but simply expelled.

One way to test whether the person is on the right amount of oil would be to put him on a scale daily and keep a close check on his weight. (This should be done routinely, in any event, when a person is on the Purification program.) If the fat is being replaced in the body, then the weight will not go up despite the intake of oil. If the body is simply assimilating the oil, with no exchange in fat tissue, the weight will increase. Such a change in weight would tend to indicate the body was simply adding new fat tissue rather than exchanging old fat tissue for new fat tissue.

EVENING PRIMROSE OIL

Evening primrose oil is the oily extract from the crushed seeds of the evening primrose plant. According to researchers, it purportedly handles various food allergies and furnishes a substance which seems to help break down dietary fat and fatty tissue. It is available in many health food stores in capsule form.

Pilots done on the use of evening primrose oil on the Purification program have shown that it appears to benefit persons with a history of an inability to metabolize fat (as evidenced by a lack of weight loss when moderately dieting), and persons with heavy drug or alcohol histories. Persons on these pilots were given six capsules (500 mg each) of evening primrose oil per day—three capsules twice a day with meals—in addition to the usual amounts of oil on the program.

Occasionally persons with a history of an inability to metabolize fat would seem to do better if the amount of evening primrose oil was increased to nine or twelve capsules per day and the regular oil dosage was reduced one tablespoon from what would be a normal dose for that person.

One medical doctor reported that evening primrose oil also seemed to assist persons who had trouble metabolizing the normal dosages of oil on the Purification program. Although this is not a common occurrence, this doctor found that when such a person was given six capsules of evening primrose oil per day along with the normal oil dosage on the program, the person was usually able to handle the oil.

ALL BODIES HAVE SOME FATTY TISSUE

All people, be they fat or thin, have some fatty tissue in the body. Some, of course, have more fat stored in their bodies than others. On this program we simply want to get rid of the fat that contains the toxic substances. We are not trying to make people lose weight.

Worth mentioning here, also, and of interest to thin people, is the fact that while toxic substances lock up mainly in fat tissue it does not mean that the person cannot have drug deposits in other tissues.

TAKING THE OIL

Some individuals reported difficulty taking the oil by itself, usually due more to the texture than to the actual taste.

As there seemed to be no reason why the oil could not be taken in orange juice or mixed with some other food of the person's choice and taken that way, this was the handling used for those persons who had difficulty getting the oil down. This gave good results, *provided* the entire dosage of oil was consumed. Others simply took the oil alone. (In taking the oil dosage mixed with other food, the exception is that one would *not* cook food in the oil and then consider that *that* was the oil ration for the day!)

WHEN TO TAKE THE OIL

On the initial program, the oil dosage was taken at the same time as one of the regular meals.

One doctor has suggested that, as the oil may coat the stomach and intestinal walls for a certain period (which could prevent the assimilation of other nutrients, especially the water-soluble vitamins), the oil is probably best taken before going to bed or at least at a different mealtime than when the vitamins and minerals are taken. This was not put to stringent test on the program and many participants did well when taking both oil and vitamins at the same meal. The suggestion is included here as a point for consideration in a case where it appears the individual is not getting the full benefit that would be expected from the recommended vitamin dosages.

ADEQUATE OIL IS ESSENTIAL

Adequate oil intake is essential to successful implementation of the program. One could not expect the desired results from the Purification program without a sufficient amount of oil on a daily basis.

And the oil *must* be pure and stored properly so that it does not become rancid.

OILS CAN GO RANCID

Apparently oils such as those used on the Purification program can go rancid after a period of time and can also go rancid if they are improperly stored or subjected to heat.

This includes combinations of soy, safflower, peanut and walnut oils, vitamin A, vitamin D, vitamin E and wheat germ oil.

According to published nutritional research, rancid fats (oils) destroy important vitamins in the body and this can eventually result in a physical condition of swollen joints or cords[3] or muscles, known as "gout." (There are recommended dietary handlings for a person who has gout in the book *Let's Get Well,* by Adelle Davis,[4] published by Harcourt Brace Jovanovich, Inc. Any person who does have what appears to be a condition of gout should consult a qualified medical practitioner.)

WHEAT GERM OIL

An example is wheat germ oil. If you look at a bottle of vitamin E you will see that it is mainly wheat germ oil. Apparently wheat germ oil, after being pressed, will only last a week before it goes rancid. Taking this oil after it has gone rancid could bring about, after exercise, agonizing cramps (or in severe cases, the condition of gout).

If a person took rancid wheat germ oil while on the Purification program he might incorrectly attribute these sore muscles to the exercise, when in actual fact it was the result of the rancidity of the oil.

RANCIDITY IN OTHER OILS

One could find oil in other places that has turned rancid—such as that contained in mayonnaise that has not been properly refrigerated.

According to Adelle Davis, some manufacturers even use rancid oils in the preparation of margarines, cooking fats and highly refined commercial vegetable oils. She recommends that one consume only cold-pressed, unrefined oils. And even these must be stored properly or they can turn rancid.

---

3. **cords:** ropelike bands of tough, white tissue which connect the muscles to the bones in the body; tendons; sinews.
4. **Adelle Davis:** (1904–1973) prominent American nutritionist.

STORAGE OF OILS

Apparently one factor that can cause these oils to go rancid is exposure to the sun or radiation. One person in charge of the Purification program in an area reported that a jar of vitamin E, left out in the sun, went rancid within a matter of days. And if a bottle of oil, or a container of oil capsules (such as those in which vitamin A, D and E are often sold), is stored for a long period of time instead of being used up, it could go rancid.

The best thing to do is to keep these oils in a refrigerator and test them periodically to ensure none of them have turned rancid.

HOW TO DETECT RANCID OIL

The simplest way to tell if an oil has gone rancid is to smell it. Rancid oil smells peculiar—it does not smell at all like the same oil when fresh.

With a bottle of oil such as that used on the Purification program (a blend of four oils), one just needs to open the bottle and smell it. And with capsules of oil, such as vitamin E capsules, you can simply poke a hole in one of the capsules and smell the oil to see if it is rancid.

OTHER FORMS

Vitamins A, D and E can be obtained in dry tablet form and it is quite okay for persons on the Purification program to take these in place of oil capsules of the specific vitamin. The advised dosage would not change.

One does, however, need to take the recommended *oil* dosage in its oil form, and this should be a blend of the four oils—soy, walnut, peanut and safflower—plus lecithin. The intake of oil is an essential part of the Purification program in order to effect the exchange of fat for fat.

With vitamins, the important point is protecting them from sunlight, heat and oxygen—therefore vitamin containers should be kept closed and stored in a refrigerator. There is no reason one could not take vitamins such as A, D and E in oil capsule form as long as they are properly stored and not permitted to go rancid.

In summary, certain oils are essential to the effectiveness of the Purification program, and thus it is vital that adequate measures are taken to ensure that none of these oils are rancid.

This is done by:

1. Proper storage of oils, including not only bottled oils but also those oils contained in capsules, such as vitamin E. Oils should be kept refrigerated and not left out in the sunlight or near any heat.

2. Oils should be checked regularly to see if they have turned rancid.

3. Any oils that are rancid should be thrown out as soon as rancidity is detected.

Research findings point to the possibility that rancid oils are a health hazard of a magnitude not previously suspected. Oils used in cooking or commercial processing of food, where they are not fresh, pure and free of rancidity, have been linked with digestive and muscular ills and even cancer.

One sees, therefore, the importance of ensuring that only fresh, nonrancid oil is used, in one's daily living as well as on the Purification program.

CHAPTER EIGHT

CALCIUM AND MAGNESIUM: THE "CAL-MAG FORMULA"

ALTHOUGH BOTH CALCIUM AND MAGNESIUM ARE included in the multimineral tablet used on the program, additional dosages of these are an integral part of the program because of their particular effectiveness in helping to handle the effects of drugs.

CALCIUM: A BASIC BUILDING BLOCK

Calcium is a must where any healing or exchange process is involved, as it is a basic building block.

More important, it is calcium that affects the nervous system.

I do not know the total relationship between calcium and toxic substances (and neither, apparently, does anyone else) but it actually exists.

The rationale back of this is that calcium in deficiency sets a person up for spasms. Nerve spasms occur in the absence of calcium; muscular spasms are caused by lack of calcium. A person who thinks he is in a state of high tension or something of the sort may simply have a calcium deficiency.

CALCIUM AND MAGNESIUM IN TANDEM

Calcium would be administered in company with magnesium. Nervous reactions are diminished with magnesium; magnesium itself has proven necessary to keep the nerves smoothed out. Both calcium and magnesium are helpful in preventing sore muscles. But they are best administered together in a specific ratio.

CALCIUM NEEDS AN ACIDIC BASE

In pairing up these two minerals, the main factor to be resolved in order to obtain positive benefit from calcium dosages was this: Calcium does not go into solution in the body and is not utilized unless it is in an acid. That is the odd thing about calcium—it has to have an acidic base in which to operate.

And magnesium is alkaline.[1]

If the system is too alkaline the calcium will not release the positive ion[2] which makes it possible for the calcium to operate in the cellular structure and go through the blood vessel walls and the intestinal walls and so forth. In other words, in an alkaline system, calcium is ineffective and inactive. Thus, some sort of resolution was required.

DEVELOPMENT OF THE "CAL-MAG FORMULA"

Working on the use of calcium and magnesium in 1973 for purposes other than the handling of drug reactions, I found a means of getting calcium into solution in the body along with magnesium so that the benefits of both could be achieved. The answer was to add vinegar, which would provide the acidic formula needed.

---

1. **alkaline:** of or like the class of substances that neutralize and are neutralized by acids.
2. **ion:** an electrically charged atom or group of atoms formed by the loss or gain of one or more electrons. A positive ion is created by electron loss, and a negative ion is created by electron gain.

The result was a solution which proved to be highly effective, which was named the "Cal-Mag Formula."

CALCIUM-MAGNESIUM RATIO

The proven ratio used in the Cal-Mag Formula is one part elemental magnesium to two parts elemental calcium.

As the Cal-Mag Formula calls for precise amounts of these elemental substances, some further explanation of these quantities should be given here.

The Cal-Mag Formula is made using the compounds calcium gluconate and magnesium carbonate. Both of these come in white, powdery form. Each is a compound of different substances. In other words, calcium gluconate contains other substances besides calcium; it is not all pure calcium but contains only a percentage of pure elemental calcium. Similarly, magnesium carbonate contains other substances besides magnesium, and includes only a percentage of pure elemental magnesium.

But it is the amount of elemental magnesium in correct ratio to the amount of elemental calcium that is important in the preparation of the Cal-Mag Formula. This does *not, not, not* mean that you use pure magnesium or pure calcium when you make Cal-Mag. Use only calcium gluconate and magnesium carbonate.

Magnesium Carbonate: The desired compound for Cal-Mag, called magnesium carbonate basic, contains 29 percent magnesium. (This compound is also sometimes called magnesium alba.)

There are different magnesium compounds with different percentages of elemental magnesium, but using any kind other than that recommended here will give varying amounts of magnesium which will violate the needed ratio of one part magnesium to two parts calcium.

It is magnesium carbonate basic, containing 29 percent elemental magnesium which is used in making Cal-Mag. And it is essential to ensure that the magnesium carbonate basic which is used is fresh, not old.

Calcium Gluconate: There is only one kind of calcium gluconate compound and 9 percent of that compound is calcium, so there is no problem in selecting the correct calcium gluconate compound for the Cal-Mag preparation.

THE CAL-MAG FORMULA

The Cal-Mag Formula, as released in the early 1970s, is repeated here.

Note, again, that the ratio is one part elemental magnesium to two parts elemental calcium. If one wants to work this out precisely, one can work out the elemental amounts. The formula below has been given for the compound amounts.

1. Put 1 level tablespoon of calcium gluconate in a normal-sized drinking glass.

2. Add ½ level teaspoon of magnesium carbonate.

3. Add 1 tablespoon of cider vinegar (at least 5 percent acidity).

4. Stir it well.

5. Add ½ glass of boiling water and stir until all the powder is dissolved and the liquid is clear. (If this doesn't occur it could be from poor grade or old magnesium carbonate.)

6. Fill the remainder of the glass with lukewarm or cold water and cover.

The solution will stay good for two days.

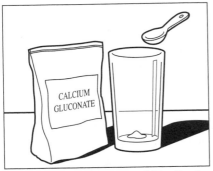

1. Put 1 level tablespoon (15 ml) of calcium gluconate in a normal-sized glass. Use a measuring spoon, not tableware.

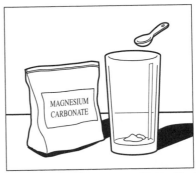

2. Add ½ level teaspoon (2.5 ml) of magnesium carbonate. Again, use a proper measuring spoon.

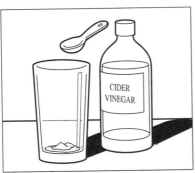

3. Add 1 tablespoon (15 ml) of cider vinegar (at least 5 percent acidity).

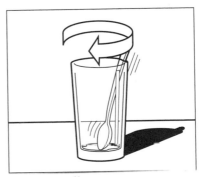

4. Stir it well.

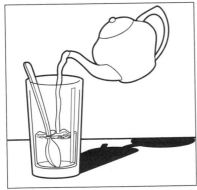

5. Add ½ glass (about 120 ml) of boiling water and stir until all the powder is dissolved and the liquid is clear.

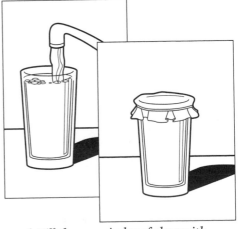

6. Fill the remainder of glass with lukewarm or cold water and cover.

Metric System Equivalents

Another statement of the quantity of each component of Cal-Mag could be made.

By the terms *tablespoon* and *teaspoon* is meant the standard household capacity measures used in the English system of weights and measures. These are precise measures and should not be confused with the eating utensils of the same names. (Besides being imprecise as measuring spoons, the names of such eating utensils mean different capacities in different parts of the world. For example, a "tablespoon" *eating utensil* in Australia is twice the size of a "tablespoon" *eating utensil* in the United States.)

For parts of the world which do not use the English system of weights and measures, the metric system equivalents will clear up any possible question as to the proportions to be used in the formula.

One tablespoon per the English system of weights and measures = 15 milliliters (14.8 ml to be exact) per the metric system.

One teaspoon per the English system of weights and measures = 5 milliliters (4.9 ml to be exact) per the metric system.

These figures can be rounded off because the differences are so slight as to be negligible, and by rounding them off they remain in correct ratio.

Substituting these metric equivalents would give a Cal-Mag Formula as follows:

1. Put 15 ml calcium gluconate in a normal-sized drinking glass.

2. Add 2.5 ml magnesium carbonate.

3. Add 15 ml of cider vinegar (at least 5 percent acidity).

4. Stir it well.

5. Add ½ glass (or about 120 ml) of boiling water and stir until all the powder is dissolved and the liquid is clear. (If this doesn't occur it could be from poor grade or old magnesium carbonate.)

6. Fill the remainder of the glass with lukewarm or cold water and cover.

Graduated cylinders with milliliter increments marked on them are available from laboratory supply houses in different sizes, so one can get accurate measures whether a single glass or a large batch of Cal-Mag is to be made.

IMPORTANT: MAKE A PALATABLE CAL-MAG

There is a warning regarding Cal-Mag. Variations from the above can produce an unsuccessful mess that can taste pretty horrible. It can be made incorrectly so that it doesn't dissolve and become the most unpalatable, ghastly stuff anybody ever fed anybody. Possibly when made incorrectly it is even unworkable.

There is also the factor that one should mix the solution in exactly the correct proportions and approach the dosage on the cautious side, as an overdose of magnesium can cause diarrhea. I doubt, however, that as much as three glasses of properly mixed Cal-Mag would bring about that condition.

Made correctly, Cal-Mag is a very clear liquid, pleasant to take and palatable. Thus the directions should be followed very explicitly, to produce a proper Cal-Mag that is both pleasant to take and beneficial.

Cal-Mag has been found to have the added benefit of balancing out the vitamin B_1 used on the program, as vitamin B_1 taken without calcium can cause serious teeth problems by setting up an imbalance of vitamins and minerals.

～

CHAPTER NINE

NIACIN, THE "EDUCATED" VITAMIN

NIACIN, AS ONE OF THE B complex vitamins, is essential to nutrition. It is so vital to the effectiveness of the Purification program that it requires some extensive mention here.

It can produce some startling, and in the end very beneficial, results when taken properly on the program along with the other necessary vitamins and minerals in sufficient and proportionate quantities and along with proper running and sweat-out.

Its effects can be quite dramatic so one should understand what niacin is and does before starting the Purification program.

NIACIN RESEARCH AND RADIATION

I conducted some research using niacin in 1950. At that time we referred to niacin as nicotinic acid and the beginning dosage used was 200 mg (milligrams).

This research was very interesting. Odd manifestations occurred when this vitamin was administered to individuals. Its most startling effect was that it would turn on, in a red flush, a sunburn on the person's body in an exact pattern of a bathing suit! These were very neat patterns. The bathing suit outline was unmistakable.

What kind of "educated vitamin" was this that caused bodies to turn on a flush exactly like a previous sunburn, showing the exact pattern of a bathing suit outline? And which left on the body a pattern of an unaffected area which had been covered by a bathing suit some years before?

Strangely, both the British and American pharmacopeias[1] advertised that this substance, nicotinic acid (niacin), turned on a flush and was therefore toxic in overdoses.

What we found in 1950 was that if the niacin was continued—in what the pharmacopeia would term "overdoses"—eventually one got no more flushes from it.

The sunburnlike flushes would eventually disappear at 200 mg, then at 500 mg they would recur but with less intensity. One might get a small reaction then at 1,000 mg for several days, after which one might administer 2,000 mg and find no more effects. The person would feel fine, his "sunburn" would be gone, and he would experience no more flush from the niacin.

But if niacin was toxic, how was it that the more you "overdosed" it the sooner you no longer experienced the sunburnlike flushes from it?

NIACIN REACTION — 1956

In 1956 I put this vitamin to use again.

At that time there was a lot of bomb testing going on and general radiation exposure. We were working with individuals who had been subjected to atomic tests, atomic accidents and, in

---

1. **pharmacopeias:** authoritative books containing lists and descriptions of drugs and medicinal products together with the standards established under law for their production, dispensation, use, etc.

at least one case, to materials that had been part of an old atomic explosion. We were engaged in salvaging these people, handling the mental image pictures, stress and upset attendant on these experiences and we succeeded.

But in 1956 niacin was reacting differently on people than it had in 1950, and the effects were more severe.

People on the research program in 1950 had experienced only past sunburn flushes. In 1956 people on the research program, while experiencing a flush, were also experiencing nausea, skin irritations, hives, colitis and other uncomfortable manifestations, on the same vitamin and in the same dosages as had been used in 1950.

The vitamin formula in use *minus* the niacin did not produce the same effect. Therefore it was obvious that it was the niacin causing these interesting manifestations.

What was this?

The behavior of niacin had been studied in 1950. In regard to sunburnlike flushes we knew what it would do—continued long enough the sunburnlike flushes seemed to discharge.

Why, in 1956, was it producing a different manifestation? The niacin or nicotinic acid hadn't changed. The bodies we were testing hadn't changed. We even tested some of the same people who had been on the research program in 1950, and they now had a different reaction to niacin. What about a case that had had all the sunburn discharged by niacin in 1950 who now, given niacin in 1956, was turning on other sorts of things? Isn't it interesting that just six years later the same vitamin, niacin, was producing an entirely different manifestation?

The *similarity* was that, with the dosages continued long enough, these new manifestations also discharged and disappeared.

The writers of the pharmacopeia or the biochemist may continue to think that niacin turns on a flush and that it will always turn on a flush in "overdoses."

But the interesting part of it is that it comes to a point where it doesn't turn on a flush. This doesn't happen by conditioning of the body; that is not what occurs. It runs something out.[2]

What does it run out? We knew, from 1950, that it ran out sunburn, which is a radiation burn. And in 1956 the symptoms those on the research program were experiencing—the nausea, vomiting, skin irritations, colitis and nasal disturbances which accompany radiation sickness—were also discharging with the administration of niacin.

Niacin in 1956 was no longer just running out sunburn. It was running out something which exactly paralleled radiation sickness.

Niacin, then, apparently seems to have a catalytic[3] effect on running out radiation exposure. It seems to give it a kick and run it through.

It will often cause a very hot flush and prickly, itchy skin, which can last up to an hour or longer. It may also bring on chills or make one feel tired.

Medical thinking has been that niacin itself turned on a flush. Something called "niacinamide" was then invented to keep from turning on this flush. Niacin all by itself does not turn on any flush.

2. **runs (something) out:** causes some unwanted mental state or condition to erase.
3. **catalytic:** causing or accelerating a change without itself (the substance causing the change) being affected.

What it starts to do is immediately run out sunburn or radiation. So the niacinamide that was invented to prevent this flush is worthless (at least for use on the Purification program).

On the Purification program, because quantities of niacin are taken and because of the heat of the sauna, it is possible that it can have the effect of discharging a certain amount, possibly not all, of the accumulated radiation in people.*

UNLEASHING DRUGS AND TOXINS

Taken in sufficient quantities niacin appears to break up and unleash LSD, marijuana and other drugs and poisons from the tissues and cells. It can rapidly release LSD crystals into the system and send a person who has taken LSD on a "trip." (One fellow who had done the earlier Sweat Program for a period of months, and who believed he had no more LSD in his system, took 100 milligrams of niacin and promptly turned on a restimulation of a full-blown LSD experience.)

Running and sweating must be done in conjunction with taking niacin to ensure the toxic substances it releases actually do get flushed out of the body.

Recently, doctors in megavitamin research have been administering niacin to get people through withdrawal symptoms or get them over bad drug kicks. They have been using enormous doses of, for example, 5,000 mg of niacin.

I have no personal knowledge that such enormous doses are necessary for handling drugs, though they well may be in some cases. It is very possible that, given the combination of all the points on the Purification program, many people would be able to handle drugs with lesser amounts of niacin, something under 5,000 mg.

*For more information on radiation, read the book *All About Radiation* by L. Ron Hubbard.

NIACIN THEORY:
RUNNING THROUGH PAST DEFICIENCIES

In theory, niacin apparently does not do anything by itself. It is simply interacting with niacin deficiencies which already exist in the cellular structure. It doesn't turn on allergies; it appears to run out allergies. Evidently anything that niacin does is the result of running out and running through past deficiencies.

Caution: The manifestations niacin produces can be quite horrifying. Some of the somatics[4] and manifestations the person may turn on are not just somatics in lots of cases, in my experience. For example, I have seen a full-blown case of skin cancer turn on and run out on niacin dosages. So it appears that a person can turn on skin cancer with this and, if that should happen, the handling, by observable fact, has been to continue the niacin until the skin cancer has run out completely. (However, in such a case, the person should see a medical doctor familiar with the Purification program.)

Other lesser manifestations that may turn on with niacin are hives, flu symptoms, gastroenteritis, aching bones, upset stomach or a fearful or terrified condition. There seems to be no limit to the variety of phenomena that may occur with niacin. If the deficiency is there to be turned on by niacin it apparently will do so with niacin.

The two vital facts here, proven by observation, are:

1. When the niacin was carried on until these things discharged they did then vanish, as they *will* do. Sometimes people get timid about it and don't finish the program, which leaves them hung up in a deficiency that

---

4. **somatics:** physical pains or discomforts of any kind. The word *somatic* means, actually, bodily or physical. Because the word *pain* has in the past led to confusion between physical pain and mental pain, *somatic* is the term used to denote physical pain or discomfort.

is creating a particular illness or manifestation. This should not be allowed to happen.

It is a matter of record that a reaction turned on by niacin will turn off where administration of niacin is continued.

2. When the niacin dosage was increased and the whole lot of the rest of the vitamins being taken was also increased proportionately, the niacin itself, taken in large amounts, did not create a vitamin deficiency.

CREATED NUTRITIONAL FAILURE

On the Purification program it is the progressive increase of the niacin dosages that determines the proportionate increase of the other vitamins and minerals.

Thus, what could slow down the Purification program and make it appear incomplete would be a nutritional failure—a failure to flank the niacin on either side by sufficient amounts of the other needed vitamins and minerals in proportion and a failure to provide food intake which included vegetables (with their vitamin and mineral content) and oil.

In such a case one would be looking at created nutritional deficiencies—not conditions which were there, necessarily, at the outset of the program.

Not knowing these things is possibly what made medics earlier believe that niacin itself had side effects. The side effects were probably somatics and manifestations of already existing deficiencies only half run out and deficiencies created by not flanking niacin with the other vitamins and minerals and oils necessary to permit a rebuild.

 ∾

NUTRITION AND DEFICIENCIES

MANY PEOPLE probably begin taking drugs because they feel terrible due to dietary deficiencies. These then progressively worsen, as the drugs *themselves* cause wholesale vitamin and mineral deficiencies. Recovery from drugs requires a full repair of these deficiencies.

Having been an early discoverer and instigator of vitamin therapy I know whereof I speak on the subject of nutritional deficiencies. Some of my work covering vitamins and deficiencies, stimulants and depressants and the field of biochemistry, goes back to the spring of 1950 and earlier. Studies made in those fields were highly contributive to evolving the Purification program.

MINERALS: KEY TO GLANDULAR INTERACTION

Between 1945 and 1973 I studied the endocrine system.[1] From this study it seemed apparent that minerals and trace minerals[2] operating in the bloodstream and circulated by other body fluids were a key to glandular interaction.

The theory is: Every gland in the body specializes in one or more minerals and, actually, that is how the glands make

---

1. **endocrine system:** the system of glands which produce one or more internal secretions that, introduced directly into the bloodstream, are carried to other parts of the body whose functions they regulate or control.
2. **trace minerals:** those minerals which have been found essential to maintaining life, even though they are found in the body in very small, i.e., "trace" amounts.

themselves interact with one another. In other words, the endocrine system of the body monitors itself apparently through minerals.

As various drugs upset the whole endocrine system, one can see that the moment one starts administering vitamins and extensive sweating and such actions, one is going to get a mineral demand in the body. Therefore, there would need to be certain mineral dosages right along with the rest of this package.

When one is conversant with the subject of nutrition and with the elements of the program, it is obvious that in the face of an unhandled vitamin or mineral deficiency the effectiveness of the procedure will suffer.

Thus, nutrition and nutritional deficiencies are both vital topics for discussion in any text on this program.

DRUGS AND TOXINS CAUSE VITAMIN BURN-UP

One of the things that toxins and drugs do is create nutritional deficiencies in the body in the form of vitamin and mineral deficiencies. A vitamin C deficiency, a B_1 deficiency, a B complex deficiency and a niacin deficiency are brought about by drugs. There may be other deficiencies caused by drugs that we are not aware of at this time. But that list is certain.

Also, alcohol, for example, depends for its effects upon the body being able to burn up B_1. When it burns up all the B_1 in the system the person goes into delirium tremens and nightmares.

In the case of other toxic substances, the probability exists that other vitamins are burned up. What we seem to have hit upon here is that LSD and other street drugs burn up not only B_1 and B complex but also create a deficiency of niacin in the body and that they possibly depend on niacin, one of the B complex vitamins, for their effect.

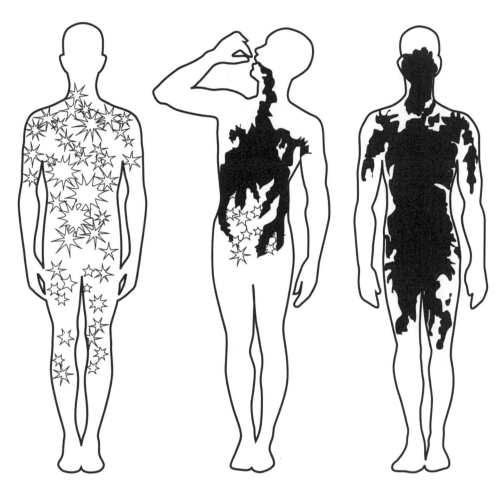

VITAMINS AND MINERALS PRESENT IN THE BODY

WHEN THE BODY IS SUBJECTED TO DRUGS AND TOXINS...

...VITAMINS AND MINERALS ARE BURNED UP

"One of the things that toxins and drugs do is create nutritional deficiencies in the body in the form of vitamin and mineral deficiencies."

In light of the discovery that toxic and drug residuals can remain in the body for years, it can be assumed that these residuals, to the degree that they are still present, might have the same and continuing effect on the body's reserves of vitamins and minerals.

DEFICIENCIES AND ILLNESS

Any vital substances on which body support depends, when too reduced or omitted from consumption, can be depended upon to result in a nonoptimum physical condition.

When very obvious, it becomes a "disease." And when less obvious and even undetected, it becomes a "not feeling good."

There is a distinct possibility that (after mental and spiritual factors) the largest contributive factor in aging is the composite of cumulative deficiencies.

Predisposition to other types of illness is in many instances occasioned by these deficiencies even when the precipitation is viral or bacterial.

Prolongation of illness is guaranteed when deficiencies remain present and unremedied.

Thus, a factor in the development of the Purification program was to handle any such deficiency with sufficient daily quantities of vitamins and minerals in addition to whatever was supplied the person through his regular meals.

The exact quantities of the substances used on the program are given in the next chapter of this book. As a part of the program itself, these then would be increased proportionately according to individual need.

ARTIFICIAL DEFICIENCIES

A vitamin or mineral does not work alone—it must be accompanied by other elements with which it combines to do its work.

For example, when one gives B_6, a complementary amount of B_2 has to be given for it to be effective. It is all very well to say that B_6 helps the nervous system and without it all sorts of things happen. But should one start giving a fellow B_6 and then wonder why nothing spectacular occurs, it is because he isn't also being given a complementary quantity of B_2.

When large dosages of certain vitamins, minerals or foodstuffs are given, an artificial deficiency can apparently be created of others not given. Increases in some elements, just by the fact of their being increased, demand increases in others. When intake of some elements is markedly increased, *balance* must be maintained by proportionately increasing others.

Lacking needed elements in one area, the body will even rob bones, muscles and tissue to obtain the missing elements.

Artificial deficiencies can be so created.

This is a principle I hit upon as early as 1950 and proved it. You can actually create a deficiency in C by administering B and calcium. All you have to do is pump those things to a fellow in very, very heavy dosages and he will develop the characteristics of C deficiency. His teeth begin to hurt. Then, when you give him C, the manifestations go away. In other words, an overdose of "X" and "Y" can apparently create a deficiency in "Z."

The reason for this is that a vitamin is making certain changes in the body and these changes, to occur fully, also require the additional vitamin. But if that additional vitamin isn't there, it gives the manifestation of being in deficiency.

The principle here is that by giving one or two vitamins in excess amount you can create a nutritional deficiency of another vitamin which isn't being given or isn't being given in enough quantity. This would apply to minerals as well.

Thus, vitamin and mineral rations would have to be taken in proportion to one another.

This theory was a major element in the development of the Purification program and remains a major element in its successful and effective delivery.

CHAPTER ELEVEN

NUTRITIONAL SUPPLEMENTS

To REPEAT THE POINT MADE in an earlier chapter, special diets and food fads are no part of this program.

What *is* part of this scene is that the person will need certain nutrition in the form of vitamins and minerals in addition to his regular meals. One follows his normal eating habits; there are no *deletions* of certain foods required. There are, however, some *additions* to the normal eating habits. These consist of, in addition to the person's regular meals:

a. Plenty of vegetables which have not been overcooked. Vegetables contain a lot of minerals and fiber as well as specific important vitamins.

b. A quantity of the recommended oil—ensuring that it is fresh—taken daily. (This would be an oil combining the four oils: soy, peanut, walnut and safflower oil, plus lecithin.)

c. Vitamin and mineral supplements in the exact dosages recommended, increased proportionately as the program progresses.

d. One to three glasses of "Cal-Mag" (the calcium-magnesium drink), daily, as advised.

e. Plenty of water and other liquids taken daily, to help flush out the system.

VITAMINS AND MINERALS

As a record of research, listed below are the approximate daily amounts of the various vitamins and minerals taken by most persons when starting the program. It is important that no one of these vitamins or minerals is taken to the exclusion of another or others.

Niacin:	100 mg (or less, depending upon individual tolerance at the start) daily.
Vitamin B complex:	approximately 2 tablets daily, each tablet containing the same amounts of B_2 and B_6.
Vitamin B_1:	250–500 mg daily, in addition to the B_1 contained in the B complex tablet.
Vitamin A:	approximately 5,000 IU daily.
Vitamin D:	approximately 400 IU daily. (This is usually taken in a capsule that is a combination of 400 IU of vitamin D and the 5,000 IU of vitamin A listed above.
Vitamin C:	approximately 250–1,000 mg daily, depending upon individual tolerance.
Vitamin E:	approximately 800 IU daily.
Multiminerals:	1 to 2 tablets daily, each containing a balanced combination of minerals.
"Cal-Mag" Formula:	at least one glass, or more as advised, daily. (The "Cal-Mag" Formula, described in Part One, Chapter 9 of this book, provides extra quantities of the minerals calcium and magnesium, and this is taken daily in addition to the daily multimineral tablets.)

Vitamin B Complex

The vitamin B complex tablet that was used in the initial research for the Purification program was one which contained:

B_1:	50 mg	Folic Acid:[1]	100 mcg
B_2:	50 mg	Biotin:[2]	50 mcg
B_6:	50 mg	Choline:[3]	50 mg
B_{12}:	50 mcg	Niacinamide:	50 mg
Pantothenic Acid:[4]	50 mg	Inositol:[5]	50 mg
PABA:[6]	50 mg		

all in a base of lecithin, parsley, rice bran, watercress and alfalfa.

The same tablet or one with similar content is still used very successfully in delivering the Purification program.

Mineral Tablet

The multimineral tablet used in the initial research was one containing the following mineral amounts per each nine tablets. In other words, one tablet would provide *only ⅑ of the following mineral amounts:*

---

1. **folic acid:** a vitamin important in the formation of red blood cells.
2. **biotin:** a vitamin which helps the body break down fats and aid in producing energy.
3. **choline:** a vitamin important to the functioning of the nervous system, the liver and the buildup of immunities.
4. **pantothenic acid:** one of the B vitamins, which is essential for cell growth.
5. **inositol:** a B vitamin related to control of cholesterol level.
6. **PABA:** an abbreviation for a vitamin called *para-amino-benzoic acid;* important in the metabolism of protein, blood cell formation, stimulation of intestinal bacteria to produce folic acid and utilization of pantothenic acid.

500 mg calcium	4 mg manganese[7]
250 mg magnesium	2 mg copper
18 mg iron	45 mg potassium (protein complex)
15 mg zinc	.225 mg iodine[8] (kelp)

In the tablet used, the minerals (with the exception of the potassium and the iodine) are "chelated" (bonded with) amino acids[9] in a base of selenium,[10] yeast, DNA,[11] RNA,[12] ginseng, alfalfa leaf flour, parsley, watercress and cabbage.

The same mineral tablet, or one with similar content or additional minerals, is still used effectively on the program.

HIGH MINERAL DOSAGES

Initially, on the program, mineral dosages were started at one to two tablets daily. Then, as the niacin and other vitamins were increased in proportion to each other, the mineral dosages were increased accordingly in increments of two to three tablets, three to four tablets, four to five tablets and five to six tablets taken daily.

7. **manganese:** a mineral important to growth, bone formation, reproduction, muscle coordination and fat and carbohydrate metabolism.

8. **iodine:** a trace mineral that is vital for the production of growth hormones. It is extracted from seawater or seaweed, called kelp, which is rich in this mineral.

9. **amino acids:** basic organic compounds which are essential to the body's breakdown and absorption of foods.

10. **selenium:** a trace mineral which helps to keep the body healthy, protect cells against oxidation and convert fat and protein to energy.

11. **DNA:** a long, twisted protein found in all living cells primarily in the nucleus. It is the key to the development of cells, as it contains the hereditary "blueprint" needed to duplicate the cell as well as patterns for the production of specific other proteins needed by the body.

12. **RNA:** abbreviation for *ribonucleic acid;* one of the compounds found in all living cells; the substance that carries out DNA's instructions for protein production. *See also* **DNA.**

Later research then indicated that much higher mineral dosages than these gave most optimum results on the program. (See Mineral Table on page 89.)

Large amounts of minerals are lost in sweating in the sauna. Thus, high, high quantities of minerals must be taken to replenish those flushed out by sweating.

Additionally, it is possible that as an individual progresses on the program there is often an improvement in the ability of the body to assimilate the minerals it needs.

PROPORTIONATE VITAMIN/MINERAL INCREASES

The tables on the next pages provide the data on how the vitamins and minerals should be increased, in ratio, as the person progresses on the program.

It is the gradient increase of niacin which monitors the gradient increase of the other vitamins and minerals given on the program. The niacin is increased correspondingly with the decrease of reaction from the niacin, as covered fully in the next chapter. Vitamins B_1 and C particularly have to keep pace with the niacin as it is increased in dosage, in order to prevent creating artificial vitamin deficiencies.

The dosages in these tables show the variations of individual tolerances encountered and the ranges of increase which have proven most effective in the majority of cases.

(see tables on following pages)

VITAMIN TABLE

This table shows proportionate vitamin increases at various stages of the program.

	Stage 1	Stage 2	Stage 3	Stage 4	Stage 5
Niacin	100 to 400 mg	500 to 1,400 mg	1,500 to 2,400 mg	2,500 to 3,400 mg	3,500 to 5,000 mg
Vitamin A	5,000 to 10,000 IU	20,000 IU	30,000 IU	50,000 IU	50,000 IU
Vitamin D	400 IU	800 IU	1,200 IU	2,000 IU	2,000 IU
Vitamin C	250 to 1,000 mg	2 to 3 gm	3 to 4 gm	4 to 5 gm	5 to 6 gm
Vitamin E	800 IU	1,200 IU	1,600 IU	2,000 IU	2,400 IU
Vitamin B complex	2 tablets	3 tablets	4 tablets	5 tablets	6 tablets
Vitamin B_1	350 to 600 mg	400 to 650 mg	450 to 700 mg	750 to 1,250 mg	800 to 1,300 mg

MINERAL TABLE

The following table shows the approximate mineral amounts now found to give best results at the various stages of vitamin increase.

	Stage 1	Stage 2	Stage 3	Stage 4	Stage 5
	(All figures in milligrams except those for Cal-Mag)				
Calcium	500 to 1,000	1,000 to 1,500	1,500 to 2,000	2,000 to 2,500	2,500 to 3,000
Magnesium	250 to 500	500 to 750	750 to 1,000	1,000 to 1,250	1,250 to 1,500
Iron	18–36	36–54	54–72	72–90	90–108
Zinc	15–30	30–45	45–60	60–75	75–90
Manganese	4–8	8–12	12–16	16–20	20–24
Copper	2–4	4–6	6–8	8–10	10–12
Potassium	45–90	90–135	135–180	180–225	225–270
Iodine	.225 to .450	.450 to .675	.675 to .900	.900 to 1.125	1.125 to 1.350
Cal-Mag	1–1½ glasses	1–2 glasses	1–2 glasses	2–3 glasses	2–3 glasses

(*Note:* The number of mineral tablets to be taken would depend upon the strength of the particular tablet used. The importance is that one gets the necessary amounts of the minerals. It has been found that large tablets may not be as easily broken down and absorbed into the body as smaller tablets may be. Thus one might not get the same amount of minerals from a large tablet as from several smaller tablets, even though the large tablet might contain the same amount of minerals.)

HOW TO READ THE TABLES

As a clarification, first of all, the figures on these tables designating points of increase (Stages 1, 2, 3, 4 and 5) do *not* refer to the first, second, third, fourth and fifth days of the program. They refer to approximate "stages" of vitamin and mineral increase (in relation to the niacin increase) that an individual goes through on the program.

On the Vitamin Table, under Stage 1, the first figure given for each vitamin shows the usual starting dosage of that vitamin used for most individuals. The range then shown under Stage 1 indicates how these starting dosages may be increased within a few days or within a week or so, depending upon the niacin reaction the person is experiencing.

On the Mineral Table, under Stage 1, the first column of figures (reading downward) gives the usual starting mineral dosages for most individuals. The range under Stage 1 shows the possible rate of mineral increase during this first phase of the program.

The same applies to the increments shown at Stages 2, 3, 4 and 5 on both tables.

Example: Person A starts the program on 100 milligrams of niacin plus the other beginning increments of vitamins, per the Vitamin Table. His beginning increments of minerals, per the Mineral Table, are approximately: calcium 500 mg; magnesium 250 mg; iron 18 mg; zinc 15 mg; manganese 4 mg; copper 2 mg; potassium 45 mg; and iodine .225 mg.

He continues with these daily dosages until the niacin effects have diminished—in his case this occurs on, let us say, the third day of the program. At that point his niacin dosage is increased to 200 mg daily, with the other daily vitamins and minerals increased proportionately, and he continues on those dosages until the niacin effects have diminished. Progressing in this way, by the seventh day of the program his vitamin and mineral dosages have been increased up to the levels given in Stage 2 of the tables. After the ninth day his vitamins and minerals may have been increased all the way up to Stage 3 as shown on the tables. And he continues in this way all the way up through the levels of dosages at Stage 5.

This varies from one individual to the next.

Person B, for example, starts on 100 mg of niacin and the accompanying vitamin and mineral dosages, and may then require a week or more to work up to the levels of vitamin and mineral dosages shown at Stage 2. He may then move rapidly through Stage 2, take another week to move through Stage 3 and actually complete the program at some point on Stage 4.

There is no rote pattern to be followed. It is totally a matter of standardly applying the data given as to when the niacin should be increased. (See Part One, Chapter 12, "Increasing the Niacin.") That is the factor that may vary widely from one individual to the next.

However, the tables given on the previous pages show the guidelines which were and are still followed for increasing the vitamin and mineral increments proportionately at the times the niacin is increased.

ADDITIONAL NOTES ON VITAMINS

It should be stressed here that individual tolerances were and always must be taken into consideration in each case.

Quantities of vitamin C especially would need to be carefully increased according to the person's tolerance of it, as too much vitamin C can result in stomach upsets or diarrhea for some people.

At the same time, it is important that the vitamin C increase keeps pace, proportionately, with the niacin increase. Records exist where vitamin C has become so deficient in a drug user that he could use up tens of thousands of milligrams of C per day before he begins to eliminate any. A severe vitamin C deficiency can result in the disease called scurvy. "Live C" from raw onions or raw potatoes is sometimes necessary in addition to synthetic vitamin C. (These were the traditional remedies for scurvy.)

Vitamins and minerals should *not* be taken on an empty stomach, as they could cause stomach burn. They should be taken after meals or, if taken between meals, with yogurt.

NIACINAMIDE

The majority of vitamin B complex tablets on the market include niacinamide in small amounts. This is the substance invented by someone to keep an individual from turning on a niacin flush. Because it does prevent a niacin flush, niacinamide is worthless.

The likelihood is that the amount of niacinamide in a B complex tablet acts only to eliminate any flush from the niacin content in that specific tablet. Results from the piloting of the Purification program, where plenty of niacin flush was experienced on different dosages of niacin itself (in combination with the flanking vitamins and minerals), indicate that the inclusion of niacinamide in the B complex had little if any effect upon the flush that resulted from the additional dosages of niacin taken. However, where a B complex tablet can be found that includes niacin rather than niacinamide, that would be the preferable tablet to use.

It is also possible to have a B complex tablet especially made up that includes actual niacin *instead of* niacinamide, in amounts equal to the B_1, B_2 and B_6 amounts, particularly if one is ordering the tablet in fairly large amounts.

Note: Where a B complex tablet that includes niacin is used, this adds that much more to the daily niacin intake and this must be taken into consideration when increasing niacin and B complex dosages.

ADDITIONAL NOTES ON MINERALS:
TRACE MINERALS

Most multiple mineral formulas include the major mineral elements required by the body but not all of the trace minerals.

"Trace" minerals are those minerals which have been found essential to maintaining life, even though they are found in the body in very small, i.e., "trace" amounts.

The main trace minerals currently include: cobalt, copper, iodine, manganese, molybdenum, zinc, selenium and chromium. Tin was also added as an essential trace mineral as late as 1970.

Nutritional researchists are the first to admit that the work in this field is very far from complete, and there will undoubtedly be other trace minerals added to the list as such research is continued.

Currently, also, there are fairly wide differences of opinion among nutritionists as to the minimum daily requirements of the various minerals and especially the trace minerals.

Minerals are found in a wide variety of foods. Natural foods, undamaged by processing, are the best sources of minerals as they exist in unprocessed foods in the combinations in which they are most effective. But minerals can also be lacking in foods grown in mineral-depleted soil. Additionally, of course, there is no one food that supplies them all.

Therefore, it may be necessary to use more than one type of multimineral tablet to ensure one is getting all of the minerals, including the trace minerals, that are required by the body.

Note: The Vitamin and Mineral Tables given on the preceding pages do not include any additional vitamins or minerals which might be needed in cases of specific deficiencies an individual might have. Any such particular deficiency would need to be determined by a medical doctor and remedied with the additional vitamin or mineral dosages recommended.

As a guideline, four of the more informative books on the subject of nutritional vitamins and minerals are the following by Adelle Davis: *Let's Get Well, Let's Eat Right to Keep Fit, Let's Cook It Right* and *Let's Have Healthy Children.*

The research data offered in this chapter is not to be construed as a recommendation of medical treatment or medication. It is given here as a record of food supplements in the form of the nutritional vitamins and minerals which were used in the development of the Purification program and which were found to be most effective in the greatest number of cases.

∾

CHAPTER TWELVE

Increasing the Niacin

Increasing Niacin and Other Vitamin Quantities

MOST PERSONS WHO HAVE DONE the Purification program started at 100 mg of niacin (some took lesser amounts at the start, depending upon tolerance) and increased the dosage as they progressed.

The best results were obtained when niacin was taken all at one time, not split up during the day. Taken with water on an empty stomach it can be very upsetting. It is found to be best taken after a meal, or with yogurt or milk.

To increase the dosage, a specific quantity of niacin was administered each day until the effect that dosage produced diminished. One would then, next day, up the dosage on a gradient, say, in amounts of 100 mg. In this way you get an overlap of the old dosage becoming useless and the new dosage being needed. This tended to speed up the action considerably when continued each time the effect of the dosage diminished.

The other vitamins would have to be increased proportionately to niacin at the same time the niacin is increased, as they are interacting in the deficiencies and more are needed.

It was found essential that C, B$_1$ and other B vitamins need to be given in ratio to the niacin being fed. In other words, as you up the niacin you would up the B_1 and the B complex. And also as niacin is upped, the vitamin C would be upped. These things would have to be kept in ratio.

HOW AND WHEN TO INCREASE THE NIACIN

Within the boundaries of the medical doctor's advice for the individual, the most workable gradient in the majority of cases observed was generally found to be starting the person on 100 mg of niacin and increasing it in increments of 100 mg until the person was up to 1,000 mg daily. A steeper gradient was then used as one went up to higher dosages. It was found that many persons could take increases of from 300 to 500 mg at one time when they reached the higher dosage ranges. Note that this does not refer to a *daily* increase, necessarily, but refers to the gradient in which the dosage was upped when an increased dosage was indicated.

Any increase was always based on individual tolerance and there were exceptions to the "generally successful gradient" described above. Certain individuals would and did require moving up on a lesser gradient according to their tolerances and according to medical advices.

On the other hand, a "grinding" phenomenon was observed where the individual:

a. held to a certain niacin dosage of, say, 500 mg day after day, until nothing whatsoever was happening

or

b. held to an increase of only 100 mg at a time in the higher ranges of niacin, even though he was getting only brief, mild results, was very able to tolerate these effects and felt he could handle a steeper gradient.

By "grinding" phenomenon is meant an effect similar to doing something over and over with the person becoming irritated and frustrated with the program and feeling he is not making the progress he could be making.

In these instances, it was observed that when the persons who could progress at a faster rate with larger niacin increases (always with the other vitamins and minerals increased in the correct ratio and by individual tolerance) did so, they went smoothly along on the program handling what did crop up.

When to introduce an increase in niacin was found to be as important as the amount of increase.

When niacin was increased:

a. after the effect of a certain dosage had *diminished* (not vanished totally)

and

b. when any *other* manifestations and restimulation which had turned on at that dosage had diminished or totally disappeared (as covered earlier in the stated procedure), good progress was made on the program on a one for one basis, providing all other points of the program were standardly being applied.

In other words, it was recognized that there would very likely be various reactions and restimulations (as covered earlier), all of which would need to be taken into consideration when niacin amounts were increased.

When this was done correctly, excellent results were obtained. Questions arising on such increases were handled according to the person's individual medical approval to do the program and further medical advices as needed.

CAUTION

It should be mentioned here that, along with this research data, reports have been received of persons found taking niacin quietly on their own without being on the Purification program and without being under any supervision, medical or otherwise, just to see what it would handle. This is not advised. It could result in artificially created deficiencies or in things turning on which are not then properly handled or resolved.

POWDER VERSUS TABLET

Some persons have reported more immediate and/or intense results when niacin was taken in powder form. This difference was most often reported by persons who had reached the higher dosages, had little or no results from a large, highly compressed tablet, and then switched to the same dosage in powder form and got more intense results.

However, several people report that they got results when taking 100, 200, 300 and 400 mg of niacin in tablets of 100 mg each; then, when 500 mg were taken in a single 500 mg tablet, nothing occurred. However, the next day, when 500 mg were taken in 5 tablets of 100 mg each, results were obtained at the 500 mg dosage.

Still others reported effective results from niacin tablets of any dosage, including the larger tablets of higher dosage.

What has been done effectively is to use tablets of 100 mg niacin each until the 1,000 mg niacin dosage is reached and to use niacin in powder form thereafter. Where this is done, or where niacin in powder form is used exclusively, the measurement must be exactly done.

The label on a powdered niacin container should carry instructions as to how to measure the powder content. With the brands that have been used, 1 teaspoon provides 3,000 mg of pure niacin.

Note: This is per the English system of weights and measures. One would need to use the standard measuring teaspoon. In areas of the world where the metric system is used (and where "teaspoon" sizes vary), an amount equivalent to a standard teaspoon measurement would be 4.9 milliliters.

CHAPTER THIRTEEN

THE END PHENOMENA OF THE PURIFICATION PROGRAM

WHAT IS MEANT BY "END PHENOMENA"?

THE END PHENOMENA of any action could be said to be those indicators which are present when the action has been fully and correctly completed.

The purpose of the Purification program is very simply to clean out and purify one's system of all the accumulated impurities such as drugs and other toxic chemical substances, e.g., food preservatives, insecticides, pesticides, etc. For someone who has taken LSD or angel dust this would include getting rid of any residual crystals from the body.

The end phenomena is reached when the individual is free of the restimulative presence of residuals of past chemicals, drugs and other toxic substances. He will no longer be feeling the effects of these impurities going into restimulation and there is usually a marked resurgence of overall sense of well-being.

NIACIN DOSAGES AT COMPLETION

Per research data, there are a number of people who have completed the program to full end phenomena on dosages under

5,000 mg of niacin. Others have gone as high as that dosage before completing.

There is no hard and fast rule laid down anywhere that says a person must work up to 5,000 mg of niacin before he is complete.

HOW TO RECOGNIZE VALID END PHENOMENA

As the person goes through the Purification program, one should be able to see an improvement in both his physical well-being and general outlook on life as he rids the system of its accumulated toxins.

Obviously if the person is still feeling the effects of past drugs or chemicals going into restimulation, the program cannot be considered complete and must be continued until all such manifestations have turned off completely.

Per research data collected, where a person was progressing well on the program one could observe him becoming more mentally alert and aware. He would start reporting exactly what was going on, what substance was turning on, what impurities and restimulations he was running out. He could usually tell if he had hit a tolerance level on a certain vitamin. All of these are valid reactions throughout the program.

As the person would run out whatever was there to turn on, the manifestations became less day by day, and he would reach a point where no further manifestations were coming up. He would look and feel remarkably better, brighter and more alert; he would have come through with good wins and he would often know and state that he felt free of toxic residuals and their associated restimulative effects (though not necessarily in those exact words), and originate on his own that he had completed the program. With all those indicators, one could be pretty sure he *had* completed it.

The amount of vitamins and mineral nutrients, exercise and sweat-out it has taken and will take to accomplish this on the Purification program is an individual matter in each case.

DRUG HISTORY AND COMPLETION

The fact of having a heavy drug history does not necessarily prolong the program, although it can do so. More important than anything else is keeping all points of the program in standardly, maintaining a well-balanced personal schedule with enough rest and nutrients, and getting in the prescribed period of exercise and sauna on a routine daily basis.

On such a schedule, persons of varying drug histories, some heavy, some light, have completed the program in eighteen to twenty days at five hours a day, reaching the end phenomena at amounts of niacin (and the flanking vitamin and mineral nutrients) which differed with different individuals. Some have done so in less time, some have taken longer.

FOLLOWING PROGRAM COMPLETION

A continuation of the vitamins, minerals, oil, vegetables and Cal-Mag, at least at the rate of the minimum recommended daily requirements in balanced amounts is wise after the program has been completed. Otherwise, a sudden cessation of such heavy vitamin dosages can produce a letdown. It is possible the person should come off on a steep gradient rather than cease abruptly. Particularly where drug damage to the brain or nerves has occurred, the body needs these things to rebuild itself. If one doesn't continue the essential nutrients there can be the apparency of a letdown.

Remember that the person has probably been leading an unhealthy life without proper nutrition, sleep or exercise. Or, even where he has kept these health factors in, he has been subjected to the pollutants and toxins which surround us daily. Thus, it would be a good idea to recommend moderate daily dietetic and exercise disciplines so he can stay healthy. Such disciplines are not therapy; they are simply a matter of good common sense.

Note that upon completion of the program, it is *not* intended that one gradiently does less of *all* the elements of the Purification program, e.g., less sauna, less exercise, less vitamins, etc., each day, tapering down to cessation of these actions.

The suggestion that *is* made is that one doesn't abruptly simply cease the extra nutrients he has been taking, but comes down from high dosages on a steep gradient to what would be a moderate normal daily requirement for him, per medical advices. And along with this, some moderate daily exercise can help him maintain good health.

Continuing all the elements of the Purification program would amount to continuing the program itself past the point of valid completion, and that is not the intention.

WHAT COMES NEXT?

Upon completion of the Purification program, the person is now in good shape to receive gains from mental or spiritual improvement programs and get optimum gain from them.

Thus, we are not looking at an endless run on the Purification program. We are seeking simply to handle the drug deposits and toxic residues in their restimulation and reinforcement of mental image pictures and vice versa. And by breaking up the balance of these two and handling the one side of it on the Purification program, we are freeing up the person to be able to handle the other side of it, the mental image picture side of it.

The latter would be accomplished on another and quite different program.

The important thing, however, is that the person is now free to accomplish it, as he is no longer caught up in the constant interaction between the mental recordings of the effects of drugs and toxins, *and* the physical effects of the residual deposits.

∾

THE PURIFICATION PROGRAM:

GUIDELINES FOR SUCCESSFUL APPLICATION

CHAPTER ONE

ADMINISTRATION OF THE PURIFICATION PROGRAM

THE PROCEDURE FOR ADMINISTRATION of the Purification program laid out in this chapter is based on the practical experience gained from the research and development of the technology of the program as well as large pilot projects during which it was delivered to some hundreds of individuals. This procedure is geared toward formalized delivery of the Purification program, however it is vital data for the individual doing the program as well. These regulations should not be taken lightly nor disregarded.

CAUTION

One may find that persons administering the program might tend to enter their own fads or hobbies into it, or, needing it themselves, avoid standard delivery of it.

Examples of this might be: giving advice based only on one's opinion or personal experience which results in alteration of the researched program procedure, hobbyhorsing some particular food fad or diet, injecting personal opinion as to the efficacy of certain vitamins to the exclusion of others, neglecting the importance of maintaining the prescribed schedule and permitting irregularities such as insufficient sleep or insufficient running or sauna time, or advising mixing the Purification program with other procedures.

It is important that those administering the program do so purely and exactly by the regulations governing such administration. If an individual reports difficulties on the program, it is essential to check to see if any such erroneous advice has been tendered by well-meaning friends or by those handling the program in a purely administrative capacity.

ORIENTING THE PARTICIPANT

To prepare an individual to participate in the Purification program the following steps are taken:

1. Inform the person that he must have medical approval to participate in the program, following a medical exam by an informed and licensed medical practitioner.

2. Brief the person on the basic theory and main elements of the program.

3. Ensure he understands the procedures to be followed, the need for keeping to a routine schedule, getting enough sleep and following the correct vitamin regimen.

4. Ensure he understands that the program does not include medication, and that the vitamins, oils and minerals taken during the program are nutrition, i.e., that they are food, not medicine or drugs.

5. Educate the person on:

   a. the need for taking plenty of liquids to replenish liquids lost during sweating in the sauna and

   b. how to prevent heat exhaustion and how to handle it should it occur.

6. Brief the person on what niacin is, what it does, and what reactions he might experience during the program and why, without making promises as to results.

7. Ensure he understands the importance of continuing the program to its completion, once started on it.

8. Get his promise to follow instructions and complete the program and not abandon it because it becomes uncomfortable or out of laziness or because he/she has other appointments or concerns.

9. Have the person sign a release which covers the above and which clearly states he is undertaking the program on his own volition after having been duly informed as to the purpose and procedure of the program and after having received medical approval to do the program.

Handling any misunderstanding the person may have before he gets started on the program and emphasizing, at the outset, the standardness with which the program must be followed is an important factor in getting a person through it smoothly.

MEDICAL APPROVAL REQUIRED

Before the participant is started on any part of the Purification program, he must first be given a medical exam and have written medical approval to do the program from an informed medical doctor.

Such an examination would include a check of the person's blood pressure, and a check for any symptoms of a weak heart or anemia.

The medical doctor also checks for any vitamin or mineral deficiencies the person may have and advises whatever vitamin and mineral supplements he should be taking to correct this, in addition to the vitamin/mineral regimen called for in the program.

Persons with physical conditions which might preclude their doing the standard Purification program (i.e., anyone who has a weak heart or anemia or even certain kidney or liver conditions) may be given a similar program to be done on a much lower gradient.

PREGNANCY AND BREAST-FEEDING

Pregnant women should not be put onto the Purification program. During pregnancy there is a certain amount of fluid exchange between the mother and the fetus, via the placenta. Toxins which might have been lying dormant could, on the program, be released.

Some of these toxins, instead of being eliminated, could be transmitted to the fetus in a flow of fluids from the mother to the unborn child. There is no reason to risk the possibility of subjecting the unborn child to the effects of such toxins which, even if present but remaining dormant, might not otherwise reach him.

Similarly, mothers who are breast-feeding their babies should not do the program until the baby is no longer being breast-fed, as toxins released could be imparted to the baby in the mother's milk.

The Purification program would be done by the mother after the birth of the child and after any final medical check which pronounced the mother in good health and capable of undertaking the program. In the case of breast-feeding, the program would only be done when the baby had been completely weaned and was on his own formula.

TESTING

A battery of tests can be done on the individual before and after the Purification program. These would include a personality test, IQ test, any available learning rate tests and others which would give a before-and-after picture of the person. Such before-and-after tests (quite in addition to any statements from the person himself) will often show up dramatic changes the person has made while on the program.

Other data taken before the participant begins the program would include, of course, a history of drugs, medicines or alcohol the person has had, his weight, blood pressure, any specific physical complaints or mental anxieties, and general details as to the state of the person's overall health.

The Program Case Supervisor *must* monitor the program carefully on a daily basis, and this is done based on what the participant himself reports as well as by actual observation of the participant, as needed.

While on the program, the person is issued his vitamins, including niacin, minerals and oil, on a daily basis, and at the end of his running and sauna time each day he himself turns in a full written report of his progress. This is done on a daily report form provided him, which contains a checklist of items to be reported on. The daily report form would call for, at the very least, the following data:

1. How long he exercised.

2. How long he sweated in the sauna.

3. What vitamins were taken and in what amounts.

4. How much niacin was taken (in milligrams).

5. What minerals were taken and in what amounts.

6. How many glasses of Cal-Mag were taken.

7. Whether salt, potassium or Bioplasma were taken and in what amounts.

8. How many glasses of water or other liquid (other than Cal-Mag) were taken.

9. Weight that day. (Include a note as to any weight gain or loss.)

10. Any somatics, restimulations, sensations, emotions, physical changes or other changes or occurrences experienced.

11. Any wins the person had on the program that day.

An individual folder must be kept for each program participant. The daily report is handed in to the Program Administrator who goes over it with the program participant to ensure that all points of the program were adhered to. The Administrator then places the report in the participant's folder and sends the folder to the Program Case Supervisor.

DAILY TIGHT SUPERVISION

The Program Case Supervisor must verify each person's daily progress and initial the person's report and any medical reports after he has inspected them. He then writes orders to correct any misapplication of any point of the program, such as skipping vitamins, not getting enough sleep, etc., as well as noting any increase in vitamin/mineral dosages that is to be made.

The folder is returned to the Program Administrator who personally takes up with the participant any changes to be made, such as increasing the niacin or other vitamin or mineral dosages.

The Administrator also carries out any orders for correcting the participant, such as getting him back onto the proper schedule if he has gone off this, ensuring any errors are handled, and handles any questions the participant may have at any particular stage of the program.

Correct administration would include ensuring the participant never exercises or goes into the sauna alone, but carries out these actions with a partner.

Tight supervision would also include having blood pressure or other checks redone at intervals during the program, as needed.

∽

CHAPTER TWO

WITHDRAWAL FROM DRUGS

THE PURIFICATION PROGRAM is not administered to those actively on drugs, though such persons need this program even more urgently, perhaps, than others. Thus, a workable withdrawal program must precede the Purification program for these individuals.

Such a program must be drugless and would include a substantial nutritional regimen.

Additionally, light counseling techniques (Objective[1] Processes), developed in the 1950s to extrovert a person's attention away from his body, have been put to effective use in helping people to get through withdrawal from drugs with a minimum of pain.

Also, quite in addition to the use of Cal-Mag in the healing and exchange processes involved in the Purification program, calcium and magnesium provide a means of helping to handle withdrawal symptoms for persons coming off drugs.

WITHDRAWAL SYMPTOMS

The most wretched part of coming off hard drugs is the reaction called withdrawal symptoms. These are the physical and

---

1. **objective:** existing outside the mind as an actual object and not merely in the mind as an idea; real; about outward things not about the thoughts and feelings of the speaker.

mental reactions to no longer taking drugs. They are ghastly. No torturer ever set up anything worse. People go into convulsions. These can be so severe that the addict becomes very afraid of them and so remains on drugs. The reaction can also produce death.

Until withdrawal procedures were developed, a drug patient had this problem:

a. Stay on drugs and be trapped and suffering from there on out.

b. Try to come off drugs and be so agonizingly ill meanwhile that he couldn't stand it.

It was a dead if you do, dead if you don't sort of problem.

Medicine did not solve it adequately. Psychotherapy certainly did not.

HANDLING WITHDRAWAL

Fortunately, at least three approaches now exist for this problem:

1. Light Objective Processes can ease the gradual withdrawal and make it possible.

2. Nutritional therapy, as sufficient vitamins and minerals assist the withdrawal.

3. Calcium and magnesium, taken in the Cal-Mag Formula.

So terrible can be withdrawal symptoms and so lacking in success have the medical and psychiatric fields been in dealing with them, that the full data on the use of the Cal-Mag Formula to counteract withdrawal symptoms should be broadly known.

The use of Cal-Mag, experimental in the early 1970s to help ease withdrawal symptoms, is now long past the experimental stage. Cal-Mag has been used very effectively during withdrawal to help ease and counteract the convulsions, muscular spasms and severe nervous reactions experienced by an addict when coming off drugs. The success of its application for withdrawal cases by drug rehabilitation centers such as Narconon has now been well established. Cal-Mag has been reported as effective in withdrawal from any drug, its effectiveness most dramatically observable with methadone and heroin cases.

Methadone attacks bone marrow and bones so one usually encounters a severe depletion of calcium in methadone users, characterized by severe pain in joints and bones, teeth problems, hair problems. Getting calcium into the system (in the acidic solution in which it can operate), along with magnesium for its effect on the nerves, helps to relieve these conditions.

It has been reported that with use of Cal-Mag, a person can be withdrawn from methadone anywhere from two weeks to three months faster than without its use. This may apply in withdrawal from other drugs as well.

Since drugs or alcohol burn up the vitamin B_1 in the system rapidly, taking a lot of B_1 daily when coming off drugs helps to avoid the convulsions which often attend this deficiency. The B_1 must, of course, be flanked with other vitamin dosages to maintain a proper balance of needed nutrients. And, accordingly, sufficient quantities of Cal-Mag are needed, both to prevent created mineral deficiencies and to work its wonders in easing and relieving the agonies accompanying withdrawal.

From 1 to 3 glasses of Cal-Mag a day, with or after meals, *replaces any tranquilizer.* It does not produce the drugged effects of tranquilizers (which are quite deadly).

As calcium and magnesium are minerals, not drugs, one is not adding to the drug effects the person is already suffering from. Rather, one is providing those minerals which are certain to be in deficiency in such cases—and helping to provide some relief from the agonizing effects of such deficiencies.

❧

CHAPTER THREE

MORE ON NUTRITION AND INDIVIDUAL SCHEDULE

T HE FOLLOWING CHAPTER CONTAINS data offered from a broad survey and review of cases in areas where the Purification program has been successfully delivered since its release.

IMPORTANCE OF NUTRITION

What showed up throughout the survey data was the importance of the daily nutritional vitamins, minerals, oil, Cal-Mag and vegetables, and the role that these nutritional elements play in handling the traumatic effects of restimulation of drugs and other toxins.

In each area it was observed that dropping out any of these supplements while on the program, skimping on them or taking them only sporadically, contrary to the program regulations, could create or intensify deficiencies which would then throw a curve into the program that would show up in any number of ways—tiring quickly, lack of energy, upset stomach, nausea, a general "not feeling good" or actually getting sick in some way, to name a few.

Any omission of these standard elements was found to interfere with the progress and purpose of the program.

Many, many cases are now reported to have successfully completed the program under close supervision on the nutritional vitamin and mineral increases within the ranges given in the original research data.

Many areas report it has also been helpful to have a good familiarity with the books on nutrition written by the late Adelle Davis mentioned earlier in this text: *Let's Eat Right to Keep Fit, Let's Get Well, Let's Cook It Right* and *Let's Have Healthy Children* (all originally published by Harcourt, Brace Jovanovich, Inc., 737 Third Avenue, New York, NY 10017). These are among the most useful and popular compilations on the subjects of diet and biochemistry which have been published to date.

DON'T IGNORE INDIVIDUAL TOLERANCES

Where individual tolerances were taken into consideration and any vitamin imbalance or deficiency handled as stipulated in the regulations set forth in the program, the ranges published from the original research were reported to be highly workable for most.

In areas where the program has been successfully delivered, the person's originations[1] regarding his tolerance for or reactions to certain vitamins were never ignored. These would always be looked into and a correct solution worked out in alignment with the theory and factors of the program as originally researched.

In reported cases where the person was having some difficulty and some nutrient imbalance was the actual cause of the upset, where the vitamins and minerals were properly adjusted as above there was invariably improvement.

1. **originations:** a coined word meaning statements or remarks volunteered by a person concerning himself, his ideas, reactions or difficulties; communications originated by the person himself.

But it was necessary to *first* determine that the person actually was *taking* the vitamins and other nutritional elements he was supposedly taking and in what amounts, or if he was taking them only sporadically.

RESPONSIBILITY OF THE PARTICIPANT

It is the responsibility of the person who has undertaken to do the program to keep those overseeing the program well informed as to his daily actions and the results.

From all the reported data, it is not unusual at certain points of the program for some to protest a bit at the large quantities of vitamins to be taken. The protest is not in regard to results or benefits but simply in regard to the quantities to get down. While the niacin was always taken all at one time, in several areas it was found most viable to take the remainder of the vitamins at various intervals during the day, after meals or with snacks. One medical doctor has suggested that absorption of the needed nutrients is better accomplished in this way. The exception to this would be where one or more of the vitamins or minerals had been specifically suggested by the physician to be taken at certain set intervals.

HIDDEN "DIET" FACTOR

Also reported was the datum that there is a hidden factor to look for if a person is having difficulty and that is the person is not eating but is going along mainly on something like vitamins and niacin and yogurt alone. Or he has made some other major change in his eating habits. This was found in one area and totally explained why the person was having trouble on the program. It was then remedied by getting the individual onto regular and balanced meals.

Verbal Exchange
Can Throw the Program Off

Departures such as those above were found quite often to come about as the result of exchange of verbal data or advice between participants on the program. This line must be watched to ensure the procedure is being followed as given, not someone else's version of it or some experimentation with it on his own.

Questions and Answers
on Individual Scheduling

Can the program be completed satisfactorily on less than five hours daily? Where circumstances honestly prevented some persons from doing the program for five hours daily, a shorter time period was piloted.

It was found that the program could be completed effectively by some cases on less than five hours per day, provided the person *is getting benefit and change* on the shorter schedule.

The shorter schedules ranged from four hours down to a minimum of two and a half hours total running and sauna time daily. This period would then be spent as follows: twenty to thirty minutes of running and the remaining two hours or so in the sauna.

The same gradients applied when the person was on or starting a two-and-a-half-hour daily schedule as on any other schedule.

The approval of the Program Case Supervisor would be obtained for one to do the program on this shorter schedule, as there are other factors which enter into it. Any medical advice or order for the person to be on the shorter schedule would need to be followed.

The program can, and in most cases has, taken longer to complete on a shortened daily schedule, but survey results show that it can be done successfully by a good many people at a minimum of two and a half hours daily *provided all other points of the program are standardly maintained.*

Is the extent of a person's drug history a factor in the time spent daily on the Purification program? Per all the research and survey data assembled thus far, which is quite considerable, the extent of drug history is definitely a factor in determining how much time daily an individual would spend on the program.

Surveys show beyond any doubt that those with heavy or even mediumly heavy drug histories benefited most from the five-hour daily schedule. This can apply to persons with heavy medical drug histories as well as to those who have had heavy street drugs.

There are reports on record of persons with heavy drug histories who, though they had done fairly well at the beginning of the program on two and a half hours a day (with some phenomena turning on and dissipating) did not begin to turn on restimulation of actual "trips" and blow through them until they were put onto a five-hour daily schedule.

Others reported that if something turned on while in the sauna they made it a point to stick carefully to the sauna time (taking short breaks as necessary for water, salt or potassium or to cool off) until the manifestation vanished, and they then came out feeling good and refreshed. These same persons reported that if they shortcut the sauna time because something uncomfortable had turned on they came out feeling bad or dull and it would then take longer to go through the manifestation.

People with very light drug histories, as well, reported feeling calmer and more alert and cheerful after a stint in the sauna which was long enough to permit them to get through any restimulation or discomfort that had turned on.

There is everything to be said for putting a person on a schedule which will permit him to handle these factors, and it was found particularly important that those with heavy or mediumly heavy drug histories were scheduled properly so that they were able to get full return from the action and wind up with the expected end phenomena.

Who determines the schedule? On any questions as to daily schedule, the Program Case Supervisor would adjudicate as to the daily time period for the individual.

In any case where the person is on a special medical program, the physician's orders regarding schedule must be adhered to.

The first consideration regarding schedule would be what is going to give the person the most gain. Wherever possible the person would do the program for five hours daily and most people going through the program have done so on that schedule.

In instances where a shorter daily schedule was actually required for best results on some individuals, the schedule was adjusted accordingly.

In cases where persons honestly had limited time, these were considered for the minimum two-and-a-half-hour daily time period, as it would be more important for them to do the program than deny it to them. But it was necessary to ensure that each person could and did make progress on the shorter daily schedule as he continued it and, if not, to get him onto the regimen that was proper for him.

Some who started at two and a half hours daily later requested to move up to the five-hour period. There have also been cases where persons on the shorter schedule were getting heavy restimulation of drugs which they could not handle on the shorter period and, when switched to the five-hour period, they did remarkably better. This can occur, apparently, with street drug or medical drug users and is something to be borne in mind. Whenever possible the heavier drug cases were put on the five-hour schedule to begin with.

Again, correct gradient was the watchword here, as in all other aspects of the program.

The supervising of cases on the program would not be done rotely but would always be done on an individual basis with the individual never pushed farther or faster than he could go. To do otherwise would be a violation of the technology of the program and a violation of the required gradients.

The successful action has been to get the person on a schedule where he is winning and getting change and able to handle what comes up, and then ensure he gets in that amount of time each day and *preferably at the same time each day.* Regularity of schedule plays a big part in completing the program smoothly and effectively.

DEPARTURES FROM SCHEDULE REGULARITY

One of the factors examined closely in the course of this survey was whether or not there was a common sauna time limit for most people (within the recommended five hours) after which the person got tired and got less return for the remainder of the period.

By "less return" is meant simply nothing happening, but the person enduring the period on a "now I am supposed to" basis even though tired and feeling he had done all he could for one day.

In those cases where the program was being carried out very standardly, there were no reports of such tiredness setting in before the five hours were up (i.e., tiredness which was due to length of time spent in the sauna). Several cases reported they experienced tiredness as part of a restimulation of drug reactions, etc., but they were able to spot it as such and blow through it within the five-hour period.

However, there were a number of reports from individuals stating they did get tired in the sauna well within the five hours and got limited or no benefit from it beyond that tiring point. The daily time limits for gain reported by these cases varied widely from person to person, the reported limits ranging from four hours down to two and a half hours or less. The individual's drug history did not seem to be a factor, as the reports came from persons whose drug histories ranged from heavy down to few or no drugs, medical or otherwise.

These cases were looked into carefully and when all the pertinent data was examined, what showed up were departures from the standard procedure of the program.

The departures found were (in order of frequency):

a. Not enough sleep.

b. Insufficient salt or potassium or Bioplasma taken while in the sauna or before running, *or* a combination of (a) and (b).

c. Dropped out vitamins that day, skimping on vitamins or minerals taking these sporadically.

d. An undetected and/or unhandled vitamin or mineral deficiency.

Correction of these factors brought about smoother progress and much improved results for these individuals.

REACTIONS

At best, any one of the above-listed factors or omissions could result in the person tiring too quickly, experiencing unnecessary discomfort, getting limited gain per hour and prolonging the program unnecessarily. The apparency would be that the program was not working when in actual fact it was not being applied standardly.

Where a person on *any* schedule reports he is tiring at a certain point and getting little or no benefit per hour spent beyond that point, one would need to determine if an adjustment of the daily time period was needed. But, as has been found, *additionally and always* one would carefully examine exactly what the person was doing on any section of the program and get any departures rectified.

Regardless of whether the person is on the maximum or minimum daily schedule, departures from other aspects of the procedure would decrease the benefits until these departures were handled.

PROGRAM INTERRUPTION

Probably the biggest single factor found in keeping the person progressing smoothly on through to successful completion of the program was regularity of the actions. This includes regularity of the exercise and sauna schedule, nutrition and sleep.

Where any one part of the procedure was being done erratically it would throw the other parts out, or give that apparency, and the effect could sometimes be quite puzzling to the Program Case Supervisor or the medical doctor and others assisting in the administration of the program.

Per firsthand observation and data collected by report and survey, where people who had otherwise been doing well began skipping a day here or there, skimping or cutting down on the daily program time or missing sleep, it usually resulted in upset of some degree. They began to report "feeling bad" or feeling "sickish" or actually getting sick following some irregularity or disruption of the routine. Where this occurred, the discomfort or upset was more severe among those with heavier drug histories.

A possible explanation of this is that the process has been interrupted and one is getting a backlogging of the drug and other toxic effects rather than a routine release of these at the same rate as when the person was on schedule. Therefore, the person could be subject to a piling up of the restimulative effects of these at a rate not easily handled by him, and this could be further compounded by any continuation of an erratic schedule.

The handling was to get the person onto or back onto a proper and predictable daily regimen and maintain it through to completion of the program.

What was stressed here was that in this, as well as all parts of the Purification program, it is a matter of the person following the normal and generally accepted rules for good health. He would then be in the best possible shape to attain the benefits which are available to him.

CHAPTER FOUR

QUESTIONS
AND ANSWERS
REGARDING PROGRAM
COMPLETION

IN THE COURSE OF THE BROAD SURVEY done several months after the Purification program was first released, certain questions and situations arose as to valid completion of the program. These are included here so that the data may be broadly known.

NIACIN REACTION AT COMPLETION

One of the most common questions posed was:

Can the program be considered complete if the person seems to have reached the end phenomena and is getting no more reaction or manifestation turning on or no other change occurring but still gets a slight result from 5,000 mg niacin?

In such a case, the person could be hung up in some error in the early stages of the program, which would show up in a full review of his Purification program history. One could do a full inspection of his folder, particularly in the area of minerals and vitamins, what effect they had, whether the dosages were standard and kept in the proper balance, whether the program had been administered and followed standardly and regularly.

The participant should be interviewed as well, and one might find departures from the regimen, such as that he "doesn't like vegetables and never eats them," he has difficulty taking the oil so he skips it, or other similar omissions.

In other words, parts of the program could have been violated and this could be showing up in the manifestation described above. If the program hasn't been done standardly throughout, one could get such a situation.

It may be that he has a deficiency which has been overlooked and not handled and thus some sort of hang-up has been created. The point here is that there could be an unhandled deficiency which won't allow a complete discharge of the toxic residues.

If the folder shows irregularities a medical check would be done to determine if a deficiency exists and, if so, to get it remedied. Getting this handled and ensuring the program is continued with all of its regulations standardly in should then bring it to successful completion.

One must not overlook the possibility, however, that the person may simply have more to do on the program.

"OVERRUN"[1]

There is another possibility, and this may be the most common, which is that the person has reached the end phenomena, has continued past it, and is now "overrunning" the action. If he has done the program standardly and did, earlier, exhibit signs of valid completion which went unnoticed and unacknowledged, the chances are that he is complete on the program despite the fact he is still getting some slight result from 5,000 mg of niacin.

1. **overrun:** the condition of continuing an action or a series of actions past the optimum point.

It is possible to overrun the program if one is not well aware of what is to be looked for in the end phenomena. There have been cases of overrun where the person was continued for some weeks at 5,000 mg (5 grams) of niacin with nothing more turning on than a very slight niacin flush effect. And there have been similar cases of overrun that occurred at less than 5,000 mg of niacin.

The possibility exists here that if the point of completion of the program (all drug and toxic residuals fully sweated out) is reached and bypassed the person could begin to dramatize[2] a niacin flush. The condition tends to hang up because it is not acknowledged or signalized to have ended. That is simply an educated guess as to one possible cause of the situation. But it is also borne out by careful study of several cases on record where bypass of the end phenomena and overrun did occur.

After the person has been on the regimen for some time, has come through good changes and is exhibiting all the indicators of being complete, carrying him on the program for six or seven days with no further effects at any dosage is really an overrun. In some of these cases it appears that 5,000 mg niacin isn't doing anything that 3,500 mg of niacin didn't do.

To repeat, completion of the program can and has been reached on dosages of 5,000 mg niacin and on dosages of lower than 5,000 mg of niacin. Once the drug and chemical residuals are handled, they're handled. The person will feel the difference. Upping the dosage does not necessarily find more to be handled. And continuing the person past the valid completion can hang the whole thing up and produce a slight effect as a dramatization, either sporadically or each time the niacin is taken.

This can then become confusing to the person himself and those supervising the program. If the overrun is continued, you will see

---

2. **dramatize:** to repeat in action what has happened to one in experience. It is a replay now of something that happened in the past.

the person become less alert or dispirited, even if slightly. His general appearance and demeanor will be a bit less bright; he may become disheartened. He may now be attempting to produce some effect that isn't there to be had and begin to feel the action is interminable. Certainly the person will feel less enthusiastic about the whole procedure and may begin to protest it. The picture now looks as if the program is incomplete, whereas what has happened is that he achieved the end phenomena, reached a point where he felt great, was getting no further manifestations of any kind (if even only for a day) and the fact was not acknowledged but bypassed. Overrun phenomena then sets in. The handling is to acknowledge the person's completion of the program and end it off.

Overrun can also occur in quite a different way. One Program Case Supervisor reported he had had cases where the person, from all indications, was complete and stated that he was complete but wanted to continue a bit longer "just to make sure." Allowed to go on, these cases promptly got into overrun phenomena. They were getting no more change and became somewhat dispirited. In each of these cases, the end phenomena had actually been reached at the point the person stated he was complete.

Thus, it appears that on the Purification program it doesn't do to continue past the point of genuine completion. Should it happen, it is handled simply by having the person spot when he *did* complete, then fully acknowledging that and ending off on the program.

Another question that has come up with some frequency is:

What would account for a person who has genuinely completed the program with no niacin reaction at 5,000 mg (or less) then a short time later getting a reaction at lower niacin dosages?

Such a later reaction, where the person *has* actually standardly completed the program to its correct end phenomena, does not mean that the program is incomplete.

To understand this reaction, one needs a good understanding of mental image pictures and how they work. The specifics of what has happened in these instances can be quite variable, but what you are looking at here in general is that there has been an environmental shift or change which produced another type of mental image picture restimulation.

To begin with, we are living in a two-pole, two-terminal universe. It takes two terminals, positive and negative, to manufacture electricity. Magnets are also an example of the two-pole aspect of this universe: Every magnet has a north pole and a south pole which attract each other and create a magnetic field. This phenomenon can be observed in the operation of the mind as well—a person's mental image pictures on their own do not react on him continually; this only occurs when a mental image picture has been restimulated by some factor in the present environment which approximates part of that mental image picture.

It takes a two-terminal situation to hang something up. On the Purification program we are looking at a dual situation: one, the actual drugs and toxic residuals in the body and two, the individual's mental image pictures of the drugs and biochemical substances and their residues and his experiences from their effects.

As discussed in an earlier chapter of this book, the two conditions hang up in perfect balance, playing against each other.

On the Purification program, we break up this balance by flushing the actual toxic deposits out of the body. With the toxic deposits gone, the hang-up between the two conditions no longer exists. This then permits the constant restimulation of the mental image pictures to cease.

But what if the person experiences a niacin reaction shortly after he has validly completed the program? What could cause such a phenomenon?

The Purification program is designed to handle the actual toxic residues which may be lodged in the tissues, which by their presence and restimulative effects could hinder or slow a person's mental and spiritual advancement.

The Purification program is *not* meant to handle the individual's mental image pictures related to drugs and toxic substances. After the program is complete, these may not necessarily be in restimulation due to the presence of toxic residuals—but they are still there and may yet be restimulated by *other* factors.

As one example of this, a person who has finished the program but who is still taking niacin daily might restimulate mental pictures of a past sunburn by spending time out in the sun. With these mental pictures active once again, he may experience a flush when he takes his daily dose of niacin.

This doesn't automatically mean that the program was not really completed. It most often simply means that a mental picture or pictures have become active—nothing to be alarmed at, as they will in most cases simply become inactive again after a short while; from three to ten days is the most commonly observed interval. These mental pictures can be dealt with effectively through Scientology counseling, but such handling is beyond the scope of the Purification program and this book.

"RABBITING"

Supervisors report there have been a few cases who "rabbited" (wanted to run away from continuing the program to completion because it was uncomfortable, or out of other considerations). These persons insisted they were complete after a very few days at low niacin dosage when little or nothing had yet turned on. But these cases were few and were easily detected and handled by bringing them to a better understanding of the program and its purpose. In two such cases where the person was mistakenly allowed to attest to completion after too brief and skimpy a run, both went into drug restimulation, which should and would have been handled routinely on the program. After full review of these cases, with medical participation, they were put back on the program and completed it properly.

Judging from reports, including the many personal reports received, by far the majority of participants are eager to experience and handle and release those conditions which can show up on the Purification program. They report drugs, medicines, anesthetics, alcohol, restimulation of various other biochemical reactions, and somatics or other manifestations turning on, discharging and vanishing, and they report them all enthusiastically and with great relief—and look for more! Such cases will often know and tell you when they've honestly reached the end phenomena.

TRYING TO HANDLE "EVERYTHING"

What also showed up on the program was the rare bird who would try or expect to handle on this program everything that had ever been wrong with him and who looked for some result above and beyond what the program is designed to accomplish. Such a case would need to be given a very thorough understanding of the program and its exact purpose, and his progress would be very carefully reviewed throughout. It is possible that with toxic residuals released from the body, other bodily conditions the person may be suffering from might then be treated with good success.

It was found important to make it real to any participant that all that is being looked for here is the person free from drug and toxic residuals and their restimulative effects, so as to make real mental and spiritual gains possible.

It is up to the Program Case Supervisor to know each case under his care, to be familiar with the progress of each case, to keep medical liaison lines in, and to know well the indicators to expect when the person has achieved the end phenomena so that it can be acknowledged and validated.

OTHER HANDLING TIPS

In successful application of the program, any bad indicators, odd or strange indicators or upset would be always picked up and handled at once.

If the person was in some heavy restimulation in the sauna and just wanted to get through it without interruption, he was not forced or badgered but permitted to go through it easily and gradually at his own rate and he would then come out the other side all right. Per reports, most people know when they are in a drug restimulation and will tell you.

In a case where the cause of the upset wasn't immediately obvious, the Program Administrator would simply sit down with the person and talk it over to find out what was going on.

What worked well was to have the participant read over all points of the program, or to have the Administrator take up each of these points with him, and the person himself would then very often spot and point out where he went off the rails. And, in most cases, he would prove to be right. It was very often found to be a matter of something having been altered or added or dropped out and this would be resolved by getting him back on the correct regimen and doing the program by the book.

If it doesn't appear to resolve, no guesswork or experimentation is done. The person must be given a medical check and any needed adjustment of his regimen then put in.

SUMMARY

In summary, it has been found that there are any number of ways in which one can depart from the correct procedure and the effects of one such departure can be similar to or appear to be similar to those of another. This can make some cases look complicated indeed—and unnecessarily so. So it has also been found that it is vital to indoctrinate the participant on the standard actions of the program at the outset and then do everything possible to preserve that standardness throughout.

CHAPTER FIVE

DRUGS: THEIR EFFECTS AND MANIFESTATIONS

VARIOUS MANIFESTATIONS TURN UP on the Purification program and these can vary widely from person to person.

Anything from an insect bite to a full-blown restimulation of an LSD trip may turn on and these simply run themselves through and vanish as the program is continued.

In order to fully understand these manifestations, it is first necessary to know what drugs really *do*.

DRUGS ARE POISONS

Drugs are essentially poisons. The degree they are taken determines the effect. A small amount acts as a stimulant. A greater amount acts as a sedative. A larger amount acts as a poison and can kill one dead. This is true of any drug. Each has a different amount at which it gives those results.

Some drugs have a direct and specific effect upon a person's mind. Marijuana, peyote, morphine, heroin, etc., apparently turn on the mental image pictures one is stuck in, and turn them on hard. LSD, originally designed for psychiatric use, can reportedly make schizophrenics out of normal people.

Though drugs are considered valuable by addicts to the degree they produce some "desirable effect," a person on drugs is dangerous to others around because he has blank periods. He has unrealities and delusions that remove him from present time.

DRUGS AND REGRESSION

Drugs tend to regress a person. That is to say, they tend to throw him out of present time and into his past. They can actually stick the person in periods of his past experiences, often past experiences with drugs, alcohol or medicine.

Drugs—LSD, marijuana, alcohol and the remainder of the long list—produce a threat to the body like any other poison. The threat is to the *body*. The being reacts by pulling in a mental image picture. Threatened with loss of a body, he pulls in a picture to put *something* there.

What he puts there is some mental image picture from the past, sometimes a combination of fancy and fact. He can do this in some cases so hard that it becomes more real (and safer, in his estimation) than his present time.

Thus, under threat he goes out of present time. (What has actually happened is that he has pulled some of his mental image pictures from the past up into present time so these are affecting him in present time. But however one wants to view this, the truth of the matter is that he is at least partially acting and thinking and feeling not out of *this* moment but out of some moment in the past in which he is now stuck.)

A person's time track is ordinarily made up of the recorded moment-to-moment events experienced as he moves along through time. But when the person on drugs has pulled in pictures from the past his time track for this period is not being made up only of present time events. Instead, what is being recorded is a composite of past events, imagination and present events.

Thus, right there before your eyes he, apparently in the same room as you are, doing the same things, is really only partially there and partially in some past event.

He *seems* to be there. But really he isn't tracking fully with present time.

What is going on, to a rational observer, is *not* what is going on to him. Thus he does not duplicate statements made by another but tries to fit them into his composite reality. In order to fit them in he has to alter them.

He may be *sure* he is helping you to *repair* the floor when in actual fact what you are doing is cleaning the floor. So his actions (which seem logical and correct to him) are actually hindering the operation in progress. Thus, when he "helps you mop the floor" he introduces chaos into the activity. Since he is *repairing* the floor, a request to "give me the mop" gets reinterpreted as "hand me the hammer." But the mop handle is larger than a hammer, so the bucket gets upset, with suds and water splashed all over the place.

That is a mild example—the kind of thing that doesn't make the headlines. But what of the accidents, the crimes, the despair that leads to all manner of tragedies that do make the headlines?

As a being can come up with an infinity of combinations, there would be an infinity of types of reactions to drugs.

What is *constant,* however, is that he is *not running in the same series of events* as others.

This can be slight, wherein the person is seen to make occasional mistakes. It can be as serious as total insanity where the events apparent to him are *completely* different than those apparent to anyone else. And it can be all grades in between.

It isn't that he doesn't know what's going on. It is that he perceives *something else* going on instead of the actual present time series of events that is going on.

PAINKILLERS

In 1969 I made a breakthrough on the action of painkillers (such as aspirin, tranquilizers, hypnotics[1] and soporifics[2]).

At that time it had never been known in chemistry or medicine (and I am not sure that it is generally known today) exactly how or why these things worked. Such compositions are derived by accidental discoveries that "such and so depresses pain."

The effects of existing compounds are not uniform in result and often have very bad side effects.

As the reason they worked was unknown, very little advance has been made in biochemistry. If the reason they worked were known and accepted, possibly chemists could develop some actual compounds which would have minimal side effects.

Pain or discomfort of a psychosomatic[3] nature comes from mental image pictures. These are unknowingly created by the person himself and they impinge or impress against the body.

By actual clinical test, the actions of aspirin and other pain depressants are to:

---

1. **hypnotics:** agents or drugs that produce sleep; sedatives.
2. **soporifics:** drugs or medicines which induce sleep.
3. **psychosomatic:** *psycho* refers to mind and *somatic* refers to body; the term psychosomatic means the mind making the body ill or illnesses which have been created physically within the body by derangement of the mind.

A. *Inhibit the ability of the being to create mental image pictures,*

and also

B. *To impede the electrical conductivity of nerve channels.*

With this, the person is rendered stupid, blank, forgetful, delusive, irresponsible. He gets into a "wooden" sort of state, unfeeling, insensitive, unable and definitely not trustworthy, a menace to his fellows, actually.

When the drugs wear off or start to wear off, the ability to create starts to return and *turns on somatics much harder.* One of the answers a person has for this is *more* drugs. To say nothing of heroin, there are, you know, aspirin addicts. The compulsion stems from a desire to get rid of the somatics and unwanted sensations again. There is also some evidence of dramatization of the pictures turned on from earlier drug taking. The being gets more and more wooden, requiring more and more quantity and more frequent use of the drug.

To paraphrase an old adage, we used to have iron men and wooden ships. We now have a drug society and wooden citizens.

If one were working on this biochemically, the least harmful pain depressant would be one that inhibited the creation of mental image pictures with minimal resulting "woodenness" or stupidity, and which was body-soluble so that it passed rapidly out of the nerves and system. There are no such biochemical preparations at this time.

The medical aspect is an understandable wish to handle pain. Doctors should press for better drugs to do this that do not have such lamentable side effects. Drug companies would be advised to do better research. The formula of least harmfulness is that given above.

BURN-UP OF VITAMIN RESERVES

Drugs can also temporarily stimulate (before they ruin them) body glands. And they can produce momentary feelings of well-being or what is known as "euphoria." Part of this is probably caused by the fact that they shut off, temporarily, the painful mental image pictures from the past.

They can also speed up the burning of reserves of vitamins. A drug or alcohol rapidly burns up the vitamin B_1 in the system. Certain drugs also burn up all available niacin and vitamin C. This speeded burn-up can also bring about a temporary feeling of well-being; it adds to the "happy state."

But when the system is out of B_1, the person becomes depressed. When the reserves are gone, the delusions called delirium tremens ("dt's") or the withdrawal symptoms that follow are nightmarish indeed.

"IF YOU'RE NUMB NOTHING CAN HURT YOU"

Drug users, from observation, are apparently sitting on the fallacy that "if you're numb nothing can hurt you." Drugs, then, are probably a defense against the physical universe.

They do block off pain and other unwanted sensations. But there is a whole sector of *desirable* sensations and drugs block off *all* sensations.

Sexually it is common for someone on drugs to be very stimulated at first. This is the "procreate before death" impulse, as drugs are a poison. But after the original sexual "kicks," the stimulation of sexual sensation becomes harder and harder to achieve. The effort to achieve it becomes obsessive while it itself is less and less satisfying. In spite of propaganda to the contrary, even sexual sensation is blocked off with drugs and this is true even after drugs have apparently heightened it for one or two times. After that it is dead, dead, dead.

EMOTION, PERCEPTION AND SOMATIC SHUT-OFF

Those who have been long and habitually on drugs, medicine or alcohol sometimes suffer from emotional, perception or somatic shut-offs. They appear anesthetized (unfeeling) and sometimes have "nothing troubling them," whereas they are in reality in a suppressed physical condition and cannot cease to take drugs or drink or medicine.

Any such case took up drugs, medicine or alcohol because of unwanted pain, sensation or misemotion.[4] The person looked on drugs, alcohol or medicine as a cure for unwanted feelings.

The only brief[5] that can be held out for drugs is that they give a short, quick oblivion from immediate agony and permit the handling of a person to effect repair. But even this is applicable only to persons who have no other system to handle their pain.

Dexterity, ability and alertness are the main things that prevent getting into painful situations and these all vanish with drugs.

So drugs set you up to get into situations which are truly disastrous and keep you that way.

DRUGS VERSUS LEARNING

Drugs impede learning. In view of all the other things drugs do, one might easily deduce this. But the statement is more than simply a deduction, it is empirical[6] fact. Learning rate—the length of time it takes someone to learn something—has been proven to

4. **misemotion:** anything that is unpleasant emotion such as antagonism, anger, fear, grief, apathy or a death feeling.
5. **brief (hold a brief for):** support or defend.
6. **empirical:** derived from or guided by experience or experiment.

be slower in drug users than others. Actual tests show that the learning rate of a person who has been on drugs is much lower than that of a person who hasn't.

Drugs, then, would prevent a person from becoming educated. Now let's weigh this against the fact that drug usage among students is not only tolerated in many schools and colleges, but some drugs are even *employed* in certain schools—one example being psychiatrists advocating and pushing the use of dangerous, addictive drugs as a means to handle what are termed "hyperactive" children.

This may, indeed, be the root of the foul-up of current education which has been so widely publicized in recent years. Teachers have been cited, in various articles in the press and other media, for failure or inability to teach. But the problem, at its root, may not be the teachers at all.

Whatever the actual statistics may be on that score, certain it is that drugs are prevalent in schools. And certain it is that drugs impede learning and thus impede education.

And a civilization that cannot be educated, that cannot learn, cannot last. This means *this* civilization will be ended unless we do something about it.

LEARNING RATE AND CRIMINALITY

Where drugs are impeding learning, discipline would also be nonfunctional.

The memory of a person who is on or has been on drugs is often such as to remove him from fear of consequences for any of his actions. The answer, one might think, is discipline. But discipline is enforced learning. If attempts to simply teach the value of ethics fail in the face of impeded learning, attempts to teach by discipline and justice actions—enforced learning—fail even harder. The person who can't learn and who is then subjected to attempts to force learning by disciplinary action simply becomes criminal.

What good does it do a government to try to get police and justice actions into effect in a society that cannot learn? Governmental threats, in a society that cannot learn, would be of no use. The society would not learn from them; therefore it wouldn't matter what measures the government took. A society that could not learn that was then subjected to attempted enforced learning would, in the end, become criminal.

MANIFESTATIONS

As a person sweats out the residual drugs in his system on the Purification program, any number of manifestations can occur. Such manifestations can be the result of one's use of or exposure to *any* chemical substance or drug which has then lodged, in whatever minute residual amount, in the cells or tissues of the body.

Incoming reports and medical case histories abound in statements from participants on the program where the person identified the reactions he was getting with past on-the-job experiences or occurrences in his life in general.

They include, for example, reports of toxic exposure to vinyl paints, insecticides, paint thinner, a wide variety of industrial chemicals, preservatives, plant sprays and the like. Some have turned on sensations which they recognize or identify with previous dental experiences, X-ray treatment, dental anesthetics such as Novocain or anesthetics for various operations, or any of the sensations accompanying various physical ills or injuries for which some type of medicine or drug was used.

This includes, of course, in no small measure, experiences with street drugs or what are now termed in some quarters "recreational" drugs, such as marijuana, cocaine, heroin, hashish, LSD, etc. If there are drug residues to be flushed out it is not uncommon for the person to experience a restimulation of the exact effects from the drug or medicine when he first took it.

Thus, one might expect to encounter manifestations related to medical or pharmaceutical chemicals, patent medicines, industrial or household chemicals as well as from any experience he may have had with hard street drugs. And this apparently can extend to any nutritional deficiency, or illness as a result of such deficiency, which has been caused by the ingestion or absorption of any of these chemical substances.

ACHES, PAINS, SOMATICS

Old injuries or old somatics may turn on, flare up for a brief spell and then vanish. These may be sharply defined and easily recognized by the individual as related to some former experience, or simply vague feelings of discomfort which are not identified as relating to any one specific illness or injury or accident. They might range from headaches, to muscular spasms, muscular aches, swellings, skin rashes, hives, bronchial symptoms or any of a number of other aches, pains or somatics.

SENSATIONS

Participants have reported the following sensations while sweating out residuals in the sauna: Light, "cloudy" feelings in the head, floating sensations, dizziness, feelings of being "spaced-out," numbness—often in the mouth and around gums or in some instances in the limbs or extremities, "hung-over" feelings, or any of the feelings accompanying street drugs.

Periods of intoxication—drunkenness—have reactivated briefly for some individuals while in the sauna, and then dissipated and vanished. Persons who have experienced radiation while living in areas of atomic bomb testings or fallout, and some who were in the armed services in Vietnam who were subject to the defoliant, Agent Orange, have done the Purification program with some very interesting results and tremendous relief reported.

SMELLS AND TASTES

Very often the person will reexperience the smell or taste of some particular substance. Some of those described by program participants are: a metallic taste, an ether-like smell, the taste of Novocain, "a bitter taste," a "medicine-like" taste, a "chemical-like" taste, a marijuana smell, to name just a few of those which have been reported.

These can show up, too, as unusual body odors emitted during periods of sweating in the sauna.

An example is one participant who had worked for some time as a lifeguard at a swimming pool containing chlorinated water. For a certain period on the program, while in the sauna, he exuded sweat with such a strong and overpowering smell of chlorine that others had to temporarily leave the sauna!

EMOTIONS

Emotions which have been shut off or suppressed may start to reappear. The person may go through emotional reactions connected with past biochemical experiences and these reactions will then dissipate. The individual may also go through a period of dullness or stupidity and, as he comes through it, become more aware. He may find he can then do actions more easily and consequences may start to take on a new meaning for him. Memory can return.

DIFFERENCES AND CHANGES IN INTENSITY

From reports based on direct observation, apparently what can happen in some cases (not all) is that the residuals of several past drugs and other chemicals (sometimes every drug or medicine the person has taken) can restimulate simultaneously and turn on heavily in the first week or ten days of the program at lower dosages of, say, up to 1,000 mg of niacin.

Others will experience these effects in a more graduated sequence, one following the other.

It doesn't always happen in an orderly fashion and in some instances it can be more severe than in others. But as the person sweats out the drug residuals and goes through any accompanying manifestations, the effects tend to become lighter and eventually no effects will show up even on the higher amounts of niacin.

A given manifestation may turn on, may or may not intensify, and then vanish wholly or partly in any one day. Then it may turn on again the following day, but less intensely. If one increases the vitamin and mineral dosage at this time, the manifestation is likely to turn on again, but it will be milder. These things don't become more and more severe day by day; they become less and less so day by day, providing the Purification program is continued properly.

At length the vitamins, minerals and other program actions no longer turn the manifestation on at all; it is gone. There is evidence that no amount of vitamin and mineral dosage above a certain final level for that individual will turn the manifestation on again.

CORRECT GRADIENT IS THE KEY

The trick is to take a proper gradient with the vitamins and mineral dosages. When these are administered in too steep a gradient a manifestation can turn on awfully hard, so the correct gradient must be kept in. And one must not "chicken out" and discontinue the program with manifestations still occurring, either.

From the original research and piloting of this program, from reports of those subsequently delivering it and from personal reports of those who have completed it, one can expect any variety of manifestations to come up, not all of them comfortable by any means. There seems to be no set limit as to the variety of effects which can appear as the toxic residuals are released.

However, where the person was on a sensible and well-kept schedule, with correct nutrient dosages and all other parts of the program followed, these manifestations would deintensify and disappear without hanging up and without undue discomfort for the person. In other words, an individual will experience the effects caused by any nutritional deficiencies as well as the restimulative effects of the toxic substances as they become active and discharge, but he comes through these periods satisfactorily on a standard program.

As long as the precautions listed earlier are well taken and the procedure followed exactly as given, the solution to any manifestation that turns on is to continue the program as outlined, with the manifestation diminishing—becoming less frequent, less intense—until it ceases altogether.

෴

Appendix

APPENDIX

A

AN EXAMINATION OF PURIFICATION PROGRAM RESULTS

SINCE 1979, WHEN L. RON HUBBARD fully developed the breakthrough he called the Purification program, two major factors—indeed trends—have been contributing to the phenomenal popularity of the program. The first is the growing public awareness of the alarming extent to which we are faced with chemical bombardment and long-term toxic and drug residue buildup in our bodies. The second factor is the program's *results.* From testimonials to scientifically controlled experiments, the benefits claimed by people from all parts of the world who have experienced the program are routinely spectacular and well worth reporting.

The following is a sampling of just some of thousands of reports from people who have completed the program.

Just as no medical claims concerning the Purification program are made, neither is any claim made regarding what the program will specifically do for any one person. However, such things as enormously increased energy, faster learning rate, new levels of mental concentration, freedom from dependence on chemicals, substantially better perception capabilities, a greater feeling of general well-being as well as improvements in a broad range of similar categories, are the types of reports that are commonplace among the tens of thousands of people who have completed the Purification program.

GETTING OFF DRUGS—FOR GOOD

The Purification program saved my life! I was totally unaware of the bad effects of drugs and toxins on my physical and mental well-being. I regretted ever having taken drugs and still felt in some ways that I'd "ruined" my full potential because I'd taken drugs when I was young, that I'd never make up the time I lost and the reserves I'd wasted being addicted to drugs.

In addition to all the incredible gains I've gotten from the Purification program, that sense of being limited by past mistakes is totally gone and my perception of my true potential is that it is limitless. M.B.

REFLECTIONS OF A FATHER ABOUT HIS SON'S DRUG PROBLEM

Four years ago, Robert came home from Marine training, very quiet and withdrawn, with no interest in work or play; no normal drive to find his way in the world. He seemed to become worse by the week, very listless and depressed; being very naive, I never thought drugs to be the problem.

After many visits to doctors and clinics, the doctors settled on prescribing the mind-bending drug, Ritalin, to "improve his way of thinking." This drug, being federally controlled, was supposed to help him in getting started on a "normal way of thinking" and doing things other "normal" people do.

Robert became addicted to this drug to the extent of hundreds of pills each week. Even though the drug was supposedly controlled, unscrupulous doctors prescribed the medication. He became a legal dope addict. In my state of mind, I called up these doctors and threatened legal action, but Robert would just find another doctor, who was anxious to make a fast dollar, and get more medication.

He became so hard to live with and so mean that he would steal from us and lie to and threaten his mother. I finally had him arrested for grand theft just to get him out of the house and in the hope of shocking him into reality. The judge let him out on probation, and he went on taking Ritalin.

We were at a breaking point and were considering having him sent to prison before he hurt himself or I hurt him (God forbid).

I was watching television one morning and saw two young men speaking about drug problems and insisting that they could help if one would just call, so I did. Then I talked to my son and we set up a meeting. So Robert went off to a center in Los Angeles that uses L. Ron Hubbard's technology. They began to work with him on a twenty-four-hour basis to help him get off drugs.

Robert began to change for the better—and oh, what a change. No more drugs. He came home on weekends, and was calm and collected and began to talk intelligently and act sanely.

Now Robert is a changed person. He no longer harasses his mother and there's no more asking for the impossible or "twisting" things to suit his way. He has really beat the drug and is well on his way to doing something worthwhile.

Our friends and others now ask how we came to have a son who is so considerate, calm and intelligent speaking. I just smile and reply that he works with a group of people in Los Angeles that help young people get started on the road of life. B.L.

LIFE-CHANGING RESULTS

In 1978 I went to my doctor for a standard physical. To my horror, I was told that I had less than two years to live. He sent me to two other doctors to verify his diagnosis and they all concurred—I had arteriosclerosis, and not much life left.

One doctor told me, "You'd better go home and write your will."

I was in despair. I was 25 years old, just newly married that year, and it suddenly appeared that all my hopes and dreams for the future were now impossibly out of reach.

I had learned about L. Ron Hubbard's Purification program and decided to do it, thinking that perhaps getting the built-up toxins out of my body would make things easier over the following months. It never occurred to me that it could help me handle the problem completely.

Three weeks later when I finished the program and went back to my doctor for another checkup he was absolutely astounded. He said that the results were impossible and that, even though two other doctors had verified his diagnosis, he must have been wrong in the first place because what had occurred was "medically impossible." There was no trace left, whatsoever, of the arteriosclerosis. It was completely gone.

I have been healthy ever since. I am happily married to the same man 23 years later, we have a wonderful 18-year old daughter, and I am achieving all of my hopes and dreams. B.W.

Before I started the Purification program my life was going downhill, fast. It was a struggle to get through each day and this caused my family a lot of suffering.

Now I feel like a new person. My whole outlook on life has changed—I have so much energy, my confidence has increased, I am more assertive, my mind is clearer and I am really happy and have an inner peace and calmness—something I have always wanted.

This program has changed my life completely and I know I will never return to the way I was. I am truly happy and able to enjoy my life. K.B.

Increasing Ability to Think Clearly

I am an attorney specializing in tax law. I have been a newscaster with a major network and am a published author.

Prior to doing the Purification program developed by L. Ron Hubbard, I had experienced the effects of toxins in my body for years. As a young girl, I had rabies shots, as well as other medical drugs. For years I have felt the effects of these poisons which I became acutely aware of while doing the program.

I never really knew how my perceptions were affected by these toxins until I got them out of my system. My ability to think clearly increased; I was sharper, brighter and generally more alert.

My hearing was poor prior to doing the program and as a result of doing the program my hearing improved. My IQ also went up ten points. This is on record as I took a test prior to doing the regimen and took one after doing the program. M.P.

More Energy and Goodwill

After doing the Purification program my migraines completely vanished. I began feeling more energetic and excited about my life, whereas before I had been extremely depressed.

I now find it is easier to read books and gain the knowledge contained in them.

My skin feels clearer and I feel "lighter" emotionally. I now have a vision of exactly what I want to do in life and have figured out how to get there.

Before, everything seemed unobtainable and unclear. The fog behind my eyes is now gone, the things that had been weighing me down and holding me back are gone and I am moving forward in life.

My mind and body are clean. I'm free from the headaches and the stuck feeling. Now I can accomplish anything in life! H.A.

FEELING BRIGHT AND ENERGETIC

I cannot believe it!!! My body is energetic, I am no longer dependent on coffee, sugar or any other stimulant. I had a terrible problem of physical ups and downs before the program and felt dependent on some type of stimulant. Now I am much more calm and relaxed, and my whole outlook on life has changed; it seems almost unbelievable. I am happier than I've ever been. This is the first time in seven years I feel like I can (and I want to) really create my future. I feel like a new person. Seven years ago was when I first had a large amount of "heavy" drugs. Actually, I never was a heavy drug user—the heaviest being marijuana, codeine for tonsillitis and Novocain. But after that point, I was never quite the same. The marijuana had a bad effect on me and those things that turned on never left . . . until now. I am calm, relaxed, ready to create and expand a new life. A.S.

It's just amazing how you can go along day after day and think you are functioning optimally when actually you are dull and not up to par at all. It is so subtle that you really don't realize what is affecting you until you do the Purification program and find out what it feels like to no longer be under the influence of anesthetics.

If anyone had told me that I was going around half-unconscious all the time I wouldn't have believed them. But that's the state I was in. Actually, the anesthetics started building up in my system from my first operation, when I had my tonsils removed as a child. They continued building up with every operation until finally it was an effort to be active. Since completing the Purification program that effort has totally gone. What a program! When you think of how many people are out there walking around feeling sort of dull and listless and just thinking they are just getting old or this and that reason for it—it's really incredible.

Prior to the Purification program I used to get periods of being very tired and I always attributed it to working too hard, etc. With the anesthetics now totally out of my system, I have not had any occurrence of this "tired old" feeling. I am bright and feel that my thinking processes are at their optimum. L.H.

Before I started the Purification program I was tired most of the time. I needed a lot of sleep and my body was always tired and out of tune. Now, after the Purification program, I always feel energetic. I get up earlier and I am always rested. My body just feels great and that has helped me a lot because I can work a lot and I don't get tired. C.D.

More Enthusiasm Toward Life

I completed the Purification program and it gave me a completely new view of life. To be honest, I never took drugs, so I didn't expect this to be as powerful as it was. But the gains I had were remarkable—I felt exhilarated, much more causative and able to think clearly. Now, I don't get upset as much as I used to, and I can think more rationally.

Things really started to go right in my own life as a result of the Purification program. And I realized just how much toxins in my environment had been affecting me. It definitely pulled me out of the fog. S.T.P.

Have you ever had the experience of driving a car with a dirty windshield? You keep straining to see, you stop and rub at it with a cloth, you just can't get it clean so you keep going hoping you'll be able to see. What a relief to get the glass really clean, so you can really see out! The Purification program is just like that, for your body. It removed chemicals and drugs from more than twenty years back that have had their unpleasant, recurring effects on me all this time. One of the best and most surprising results of this program is that my nearsightedness has actually improved—I have to get less powerful lenses for my eyes. It's like getting a new body. H.K.

My vision has become brighter and improved. My taste is much sharper and some things even taste completely different now, through a purified body. I recommend the Purification program HIGHLY to ANYONE. M.C.

I just completed the Purification program and I feel fantastic. My body moves easily instead of being sluggish. I no longer have those "pictures" which used to confuse me. Now they're gone and there's nothing between me and what I observe. I am happier and more self-confident. L.M.

THINK AND UNDERSTAND THINGS FASTER

Since having finished the Purification program my ability to study has increased about double plus. My ability to spot and handle things I don't understand has gotten very acute. There is a lot less hesitancy to dive into some theory or do some practical drill that I have never done before or am not familiar with, due to the fact of seeing things more clearly and just seeming to have a quicker ability to compute and comprehend correctly what it actually is I am studying. L.W.

It is much easier to concentrate on the study materials. My ability to understand what I've read is much increased. I can picture what the author is saying, making it much easier to read. V.L.

Before doing the Purification program, I was a medium student. I would study and get something out of it, but sometimes it was hard to get a concept or to understand a subject easily and understand every aspect of that subject. With the program now done, I feel I'm better at studying. It's easy for me to understand anything. I grasp the meanings of things in an instant. I even feel more intelligent and I have become one of the best students on my courses. C.D.

Side Effects from Past Drugs Gone

I recently completed the Purification program and I must say it was the best cleansing program I've ever been on. Before doing the program I had been on diets, done exercise programs and fasted in an effort to cleanse my body of the toxins and impurities. But on all these programs, the residual deposits of drugs in the body were never addressed and so I continued to be affected by them. For instance, I'd go running and jog loose some residual effects of sodium pentothal from a previous tooth extraction and I'd feel faint for a few seconds at a time intermittently over the next few weeks. On the Purification program my circulation improved greatly and I sweated out all residual drug deposits. The proof of this to me is how I feel now. None of the previous "side effects" of drugs occur anymore when I exercise and am heavily active! I feel really healthy! M.J.M.

About six years ago I had an asthma attack though I hadn't had any symptoms of it since I was a baby. I thought it would just go away but it was getting worse and worse every year and I had three trips to the hospital and Emergency clinic to handle some serious (and frightening) asthma attacks.

I was becoming more and more dependent on asthma medication and I was having to reduce my work schedule to get more sleep, etc.

I then found out about the Purification program and how it would get rid of harmful effects of drugs and medications.

While doing the program I kept forgetting to take my asthma medications (something I would never have done before) and I kept waiting for some wheezing or labored breathing to occur as a result, but nothing happened. I increased the strenuousness of my exercises and still no asthma symptoms occurred. It slowly began to dawn on me that my asthma was gone! I was doing all the things that would have caused it to flare up in the past, but nothing was happening!

I realized that I had handled the toxins in my body so there was nothing to restimulate the asthma.

I can't express my relief and happiness and my sincere and undying gratitude to L. Ron Hubbard for this technology. It is miraculous. J.L.C.

Physically I feel much better since being on the Purification program. My appetite is under my control. Before, I would go on eating binges. Now I don't. I eat what I want but it's not too much and I eat more healthful foods. My skin, which broke out badly the first time I came off drugs, has cleared up a lot. It's now on the road to recovery and I feel much better about myself and my body. S.U.

FACING LIFE WITHOUT DRUGS

My Purification program is finally complete and without a doubt I'd call it a complete success. I originally did it because I wanted to kick the drug scene, as well as my inability to do good in school. What I've gotten out of it is much, much more. I can now face up to everyday life and its problems without having to depend on a "crutch" to get me through the day. I've known for a long time that for me to get ahead in this world, I had to get out and do it myself, because nobody is going to do it for me. That's where drugs hurt me. They kept me from being able to do it on my own. Now I've finally escaped from that prison and can go on living my life the way it should be. Until now I hadn't even looked past college. Now, I'm looking way ahead to what I have to do and my dreams and aspirations. I enjoy being "straight" now, whereas before I hated it. N.S.

I have just participated in a miracle. I would never have believed that I would ever feel this good again. The Purification program saved my life, my soul, and in addition has made me a better human being. T.K.

Having completed the Purification program I feel fantastic. I feel like a teenager. I know my body is clean. I feel lighter and it's great to move my body with no effort. I've realized that this is the way my body is supposed to feel and I don't want to put anything into it to make it dirty. My mind is also bright and clear. I now can remember things. D.M.

RADIATION: CASE HISTORIES

CHERNOBYL

On an early spring morning in April 1986 workers at the Chernobyl nuclear power plant were conducting tests. While in the process of bringing reactor power levels down using a highly unusual and risky procedure, they lost control of the reaction. As the out-of-control nuclear reaction continued, steam pressure in the reactor climbed to extremely high levels, causing the protective cladding of the fuel to disintegrate. Free of its covering, the melting fuel reacted with the steam to form oxygen and hydrogen gas, both extremely explosive. A steam explosion, which ruptured the reactor vessel, was followed immediately by a hydrogen/oxygen explosion, which disintegrated the reactor and demolished the containment building, releasing huge quantities of radioactivity into the atmosphere.

The damage from the explosions destroyed the reactor, resulting in failure of all containment systems. Radioactivity from the explosion began to blow north, where it was detected first in Finland. Eventually, the rest of the world learned of the disaster.

There were 13 deaths due to radiation exposure received on the night of the accident. In all, 38 persons died as a result of Acute Radiation Syndrome. 135,000 residents within a 10-mile radius had to be evacuated. Today, several million people live on soil contaminated as a result of the disaster. Some projections suggest that 20,000–40,000 persons will die prematurely from radiation-induced cancer.

One of the most heavily affected areas in Russia is Bryansk, in the direct path of the radiation plume. Bryansk experienced radiation levels 100–1,000 times greater than acceptable release limits in the US. Many of those contaminated were children. In cooperation with the Russian government, 14 children, ages 10–15, were put through the detoxification program. To some extent, cesium-137 is naturally and gradually eliminated from the body. The younger the child, the faster the excretion rate. Cesium levels were measured when the children arrived for detoxification. After a waiting period of ten days, they began the program. All of the children experienced reductions beyond those predicted by normal excretion rates, with some achieving total elimination.

When faced with industrial or environmental accidents, safety professionals need treatment that is simple, economic and can be set up and administered quickly. In my experience, the Hubbard detoxification procedure is one of the few methods that meets these criteria. J.B.

X-RAY EXPOSURE

Reports have also been received which detail the results of the Purification program on people with a history of radiation exposure. One physician reported this when he completed the program:

Prior to starting the Purification program, I had a history of moderately heavy radiation exposure. This consisted of long periods of sun exposure through childhood and college and frequent X-ray exposure from working around X-ray machines with patients for some seven-odd years. I had no physical problems or complaints upon starting the Purification program. My drug history had been very light. During the program I had several episodes of extreme flush, splotchy rashes accompanied by nausea and a very solid, wooden feeling.

At times, there was an electrical kind of discharge from the body especially to the arms and hands. Interestingly enough, after the program I realized several low-grade sensations or pains that I previously had ignored were gone. Small things, like occasionally unexplained nausea or mild aches in the muscles and joints. Consequently some attention is freed from the body and the above sensations and pains have not particularly reoccurred in the two years since finishing the program. From my viewpoint as a physician, this raises several questions on what effects low-grade radiation of different types over a lifetime can have on a being or his body—probably more significant than is currently recognized. G.D.

NUCLEAR REACTORS

One individual worked on a contamination clean-up crew at the atomic research center in Hanford, Washington. He had worked inside nuclear reactors and once reported inhaling highly contaminated dust. He said he recalled working in one specific area that was so "hot" he was only permitted one minute of work in the area per day. Other areas he'd worked in had longer "burn-out" time such as ten minutes or thirty minutes. He later underwent the Purification program.

Before the program I felt "massy" around the head. I thought I was doing okay but I knew it wasn't quite right. I felt as though something needed to be handled. While doing the program I went through periods of blankness for days. I just couldn't seem to remember things. Also, I went through about one week of not being able to catch my breath. You know, I didn't even realize I had had a problem with it, but now I can recall shortness of breath while mountain climbing but only when the weather was hot. After the program, I am in great shape. I feel sharp, alert and ready to face life. I sure do feel better about life and myself now. B.H.

ATOMIC TESTING

Two particular cases focused on the US atomic testing in the 1950s.

One such case involves a person who grew up in Utah and as a child was exposed to the radioactive fallout from the US government's nuclear tests in neighboring Nevada. He completed the Purification program in February of 1980 and described some of his experiences:

It should be noted what happened one night in the sauna. After I had been in there for some three hours I turned on a tremendous amount of radiation. There was no redness with the niacin, merely the tremendous heat and pain I felt when I got a good deal of radiation from atomic blasts in 1953. I almost died from radiation burns at that time. I received a great deal of atomic radiation from drinking water that had been filled with fallout. In the sauna I experienced the full return of that moment. I felt the grief and the anger and the pain and the swelling of the face and the blisters and the pain through to the bones. I then went back into the sauna and was able to "blow off" a good deal of this feeling by further sauna exposure.

I feel I have now run out all the drugs and the extreme radiation that I was exposed to in this lifetime. I regained my affinity for people and have a greater love and tolerance for them as a result of the drugs being removed. There have been times on this program when I felt such exhilaration and felt the way I felt when I was a kid.

My friends that I grew up with have not been so fortunate. The atomic tests or the fallout from those tests in Nevada, falling on Utah, have done such a great deal of damage to so many lives. Some of my friends in Utah are dead as a result of those tests. My life would have gone by the boards if I had not had this program. There is a deep sense of gratitude to L. Ron Hubbard for this program. H.J.

Another case was a man who was one of 2,100 marines who received orders to participate in nuclear weapons testing at the Nevada test site. He witnessed two atomic detonations in June and July of 1957. The second explosion, 77 kilotons, was the largest atmospheric blast test ever conducted within the continental limits of the United States. He was in an open trench 3 miles from the explosion. Shortly afterwards, he was sent in to within 300 yards of "ground zero." He once described to a newspaper reporter his recollection of the first blast.

We were told to bend down in the ditch and cover our eyes with our forearms. When that blast went off, I could see the bone in my arm through my closed eyes. We were thrown back and forth in that ditch. It was like a stampede of cattle went over us. The force and heat were tremendous. We had burns on the back of our necks. We weren't prepared ahead of time for any of this. We were as innocent as children until that bomb lit up the sky as bright as day and I turned to see a manikin behind me with its face on fire.

In 1978, he started feeling sick. He said he went to thirty-six doctors but they couldn't determine what was wrong with him. Years later people had told him about the program and in 1983 he decided to try it. He reported his observations:

My improvements were multifaceted. When I began this program I had reached the point where I felt that a return to well-being was highly improbable if not impossible. During the first thirteen to fourteen days of the program I continued to believe that improvement was out of the question for me. And then—WHAMO! Something miraculous happened! Damned if I didn't begin to feel better. A little better at first in subtle yet noticeable ways. For instance, my stamina increased; my feelings of tiredness began to dissipate slowly and grudgingly. Towards the end of the program I realized that I had more vitality than at any time in the last seven or eight years. Emotionally, I felt up. Depression lifted and I could once again feel exhilaration when such moments occurred. There is new hope for radiation victims! I'm the living proof of it! T.S.

CHEMICAL EXPOSURE:
AN OCCUPATIONAL CASE HISTORY

One which was particularly noteworthy involved a woman who went to her physician complaining of chemical exposure. Among her complaints were a constant feeling of tiredness, skin problems, and a general feeling of "feeling terrible all the time." She said she was exposed to toxic chemicals during her employment at an electronics manufacturing company. Each night she cleaned filters in a system designed to entrap soot and other particles. She washed them with already contaminated water which she described as blackish and oily.

After several interviews with medical experts, an occupational health specialist suggested she undergo L. Ron Hubbard's program under his care. She decided to do so.

Four days into the program she reported "black junk" coming from her pores that resembled water she used at work. This was noted on the arms, neck, face. The outpouring of this black, oily material continued throughout the program though in lesser and lesser amounts until she was done.

Her physician, a diplomate in occupational medicine and a medical doctor for over twenty years, who also holds a Master of Public Health degree, reported his observations which included the following:

I saw her for a post-treatment evaluation. Subjectively, she was feeling fine. She noted specifically a great increase in her energy level, felt that her eyesight was much improved, that her skin had cleared considerably, including improvement in the gum problems that she had noted, hair less oily and other subjective improvements such as better outlook on life, decrease in the lymph gland swellings, and a general improvement in her feeling of well-being.

In summary, [this patient] has had a very successful response to the Hubbard program of detoxification. She feels well and is ready to return to full employment of any type which she can find.

I am convinced that the Hubbard program of detoxification is the only mechanism now available to rid the body of fat-soluble toxic substances. I believe this case will amply demonstrate that it is, indeed, effective. D.R.

AGENT ORANGE: CASE HISTORIES

For several years, one of the most controversial if not explosive toxic contamination topics has been Agent Orange, the herbicide-defoliant sprayed by United States military aircraft in the jungles of Vietnam. The key ingredient in Agent Orange is dioxin, a deadly chemical reported to store in body tissues and which even in minute quantities can cause serious adverse health effects.

There have been several cases where individuals who claimed they had been exposed to Agent Orange completed the Purification program. While no facility delivering the Purification program makes claims for the elimination of Agent Orange symptoms, the following reports are examples that do offer great hope:

Prior to the Purification program something was wrong. Objectively I was acting analytically but from time to time subjectively I would experience psychosis and neurosis in specific areas of my life which tended to hamper me as a being. I am an ex-Marine who had fought in the Vietnam War from 1968 to 1969.

Besides the constant fighting I was also exposed to deadly poisonous gases and toxins, especially Agent Orange and some sort of nerve gas while in the service and in the Vietnam War. Through the Purification program these toxins were fully flushed out. They had actually prevented me from thinking straight and logically; inhibited my perceptions and control of my body. Boy was I ever in for a surprise during the program and after completion!

I literally erased an incident which had me stuck on "the track,"[1] dramatizing it in present time, that I wasn't aware of. I had

---

1. **track:** short for *time track,* the consecutive recording of mental image pictures which accumulates through a person's existence.

considered my environment dangerous—I mean really dangerous, as it was in the jungles of South Vietnam. But would you believe that I was still "in" South Vietnam though I left it in 1969? I was fully brought out of it as well as oriented to my present environment by the Purification program.

It really undercut everything, I mean, these were such very simple actions to do but powerful insofar as the results and gains I had. Both objectively and subjectively the Purification program has changed my life, my physical well-being and my attitude towards a much better existence of survival. I no longer have to look over my shoulder for "the enemy" (which wasn't there) or walk carefully through any grassy areas (looking for land mines which don't exist) so that I can live another day.

It has opened a door for me—a door through which I can experience life. My physical being is much better insofar as its coloration and pigment. Many other people have commented on how healthy I look. I feel healthy and I am aware that I am in control of my body which had been hampered prior to the Purification program by those toxins, especially Agent Orange. As a Vietnam vet, I can say that life is definitely worthwhile to experience and create. There is hope for those Vietnam vets who are still in the Vietnam War syndrome after being out of the war. W.B.

Here is another report, from a man who enlisted in the Army in 1962. In 1964, he was airlifted to Saigon, Vietnam, and from there on to Thailand. In a legally sworn affidavit, he tells his story:

During that year, October 1964 to October 1965, I noticed that aircrafts would sometimes spray the jungle just outside the base I was on. During one of these sprayings the wind was blowing in my direction and some of the spray mist landed on my skin in the area of my neck and upper chest. A corporal had told me that the spraying was done to keep the jungle from growing too high.

Within a week or so of the spray coming in contact with my skin, I had developed open sores that bled slightly. These were just in the area that the spray mist had touched.

I went to the field hospital to have this condition checked as I was afraid of what was happening. These sores did not heal at all and seemed to be getting worse. I was examined at that field hospital and the sores were diagnosed as acne; very acute acne. I was told to wash better and was given some peroxide to use to clean the sores. I did exactly as told and the sores got deeper. One was so deep that I could put a "Q-Tip" all the way into it and past the cotton swab on the end of the "Q-Tip." I must say I felt very apathetic about this condition.

I was due for return to the United States and release from the service in October 1965. I went again to the field hospital for my medical release and again was told I did not wash good enough and still had the acne. I was not and am not a doctor so I believed what I was told and took my release and returned to the United States where I was discharged.

From October 1965 until sometime in 1978 I had these sores. They were always open and sometimes bleeding slightly. Sometimes I would also be upset mentally.

During 1978 I was a parishioner at the Church of Scientology Mission of Fort Lauderdale, Florida. One of the services offered at the mission at the time was a program designed to handle the harmful effects of drug residues stored in the body. This program was called the "Sweat Program."

Within two weeks after starting the "Sweat Program" besides the spiritual benefit I was feeling, the sores had cleared up and I felt good again although the sores had not totally disappeared.

The "Sweat Program" was later refined and improved upon and was replaced by the Purification program. During 1981 I did the Purification program and the sores healed totally. It was while on this program that I finally realized that the sores came from the Agent Orange that I was exposed to in 1965. R.T.

The experience related above was not unique. Another man served with a Marine Air Traffic Control Unit in Vietnam from August 1967 to August 1968. He was sure he was exposed to Agent Orange as they sprayed the defoliant within two or three miles of his base.

Upon returning from Vietnam, I had continual problems with rashes all over my body. I later found out this is termed chloracne. I also had liver problems, continuous headaches (migraines) and an inability to tolerate much liquor without getting ill. Additionally, my wife had two miscarriages and had since not been able to get pregnant.

About a year ago, I completed the Purification program. I am no longer troubled with the chloracne; I still have white spots on my body where I had had rashes in the past. I seldom have headaches and the headaches I do have are rarely of the intensity of the ones I previously had.

My wife is now pregnant again and is over four months along. The longest she was able to carry a pregnancy in the past was less than three months. I attribute these changes in my physical health directly to having done L. Ron Hubbard's Purification program. S.H.

This ex-Marine wrote his report in December of 1981. The child he was expecting at the time was born healthy, a baby boy. And his family has grown since then, as the couple went on to have another child, a healthy baby girl.

SCIENTIFIC TESTING

Three years after the program was released, it was independently tested on a group of people who were contaminated with a fire-retardant chemical (polybrominated biphenyls or PBBs).* They were residents of the state of Michigan where millions of people were exposed to the chemical during a massive agricultural contamination in the early 1970s. Previous studies had already established that it takes ten to twenty years or more for the stored residues of PBBs and similar chemicals, such as PCBs (polychlorinated biphenyls, components which are found in industrial coolants) to be reduced naturally by just one half. In light of this, the group of researchers designed a study to measure their fat levels of PBBs, PCBs and several other chemicals before, immediately after, and four months following Purification program. The results were quite startling.

---

*In the summer of 1973, toxic fire-retardant chemicals were accidentally added to livestock feed in Michigan. An extensive study by researchers from Mount Sinai School of Medicine in New York City indicated that even five years after the accident, nearly all of the state's population had been contaminated with polybrominated biphenyls or PBBs. The contamination incident is detailed in several publications. Some suggested ones include: *PBB: An American Tragedy,* by Erwin Chen, Prentice-Hall, 1979; *The Contamination Crisis in Michigan: Polybrominated Biphenyls, A Report From The Senate Special Investigation Committee,* Michigan State Senate, July 1975.

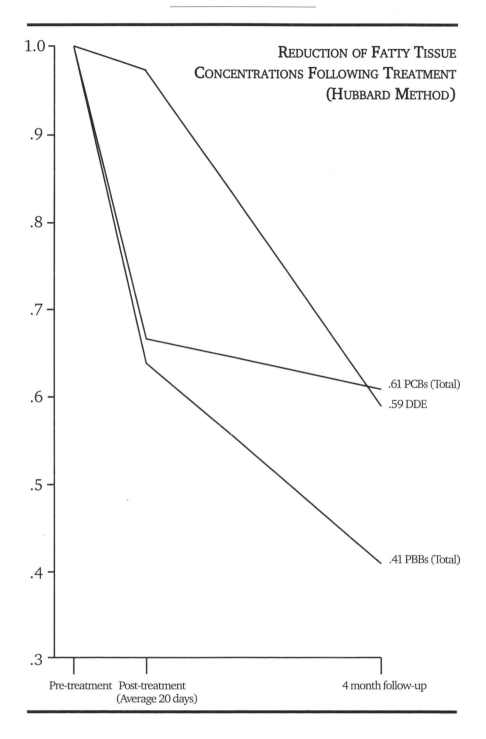

Reduction of Fatty Tissue
Concentrations Following Treatment
(Hubbard Method)

.61 PCBs (Total)
.59 DDE
.41 PBBs (Total)

Pre-treatment Post-treatment
(Average 20 days)   4 month follow-up

REDUCTION OF TOXIC CHEMICAL LEVELS IN THE BODY

The study group reported that the Purification program brought about an immediate average reduction of approximately 20 percent for 16 different chemicals studied. The results of a four-month follow-up examination revealed an average reduction of over 40 percent for all chemicals. The fact that the chemical levels continued to go down after the program was completed was a phenomenon found in other studies as well. In 1984, a physician reported in the journal, *Clinical Research,* his findings after testing the fat of a person who underwent the program. At the end of 53 days, he reported that the tissue level of a DDT-related chemical (DDE) was reduced by 29 percent. At the end of 250 days—long after his patient had completed the Purification program—the DDE level had been reduced by 97 percent.

Writing in the May 1984 magazine of the US National Safety Council, researcher Dr. Max Ben said, "Given the fact that more than 20 million Americans work with chemicals known to be toxic to the nervous system and other parts of the body, the potential benefits of detoxification techniques such as that developed by Hubbard are immense. If, as the Hubbard regimen seems to indicate, chemical toxins can be removed safely and effectively from the body, then it may be possible to resolve the entire problem of human contamination and chemically related disease."

CONCLUSION

The intention in this appendix has not been to offer promises of cures or claims but a relative handful of examples of what thousands of people have experienced when undergoing the Purification program as described in this book. It would not be difficult to fill an entire book with such reports—the benefits people report cover an enormous range of improvement categories. So while no medical claims are, or are ever made, for the Purification program, we have selected case reports which provide a broad view of persons who have undergone the program and the types of phenomena which have been reported by them.

The Editors

WHERE TO DO THE PURIFICATION PROGRAM

CHURCHES HAVE EXISTED since the dawn of man with the purpose of assisting people in their aspirations toward happier and more fulfilling lives.

With the escalation of the drug problem and its disastrous consequences both for the individual and the society, offering a service which can help a person overcome and reverse the damage caused by drugs and toxins becomes a vital necessity to fulfilling such a purpose.

Since 1980, Churches of Scientology have been offering just such a service—L. Ron Hubbard's Purification program. Tens of thousands of people have successfully completed the program at Scientology churches and organizations. The statements of those who have finished the program are full of wonder at the improvements in themselves and praise for the man who researched and developed the program—L. Ron Hubbard.

Mr. Hubbard's life's work was devoted to developing a technology with which to help people attain spiritual awareness and freedom. As he said in an article called *My Philosophy:*

"I like to help others and count it as my greatest pleasure in life to see a person free himself of the shadows which darken his days.

"These shadows look so thick to him, and weigh him down so, that when he finds they are *shadows and that he can see through them, walk through them and be again in the sun, he is enormously delighted. And I am afraid I am just as delighted as he is."*

There is no reason for *anyone* to be trapped in the shadows of the effects of drugs and toxins.

Scientology churches and organizations are fully set up to deliver the Purification program, with technical personnel thoroughly trained in the exact application and supervision of the program. Every day, people walk into Scientology organizations around the world and start the Purification program. These are people from all walks of life: former drug addicts, businessmen, celebrities, housewives. Their reasons for starting the program differ, but in doing the program each one is taking a major step on the road to true freedom and personal ability.

You can do the Purification program at a Scientology church or organization in your own area. A list of Scientology organizations is included at the back of this book—contact the one nearest you.

W H E R E   T O   D O   T H E
P U R I F I C A T I O N   P R O G R A M

The Purification program provides a means by which an individual, a group and a whole society might take the first step up toward a toxin-free, drug-free civilization.

It is offered here as an invitation to start living!

The Editors

GLOSSARY

GLOSSARY

additive: a thing which has been added. This usually has a bad meaning in that an additive is said to be something needless or harmful which has been done in addition to standard procedure. Additive normally means a departure from standard procedure. PART ONE, CHAPTER 6, #1

alkaline: of or like the class of substances that neutralize and are neutralized by acids. PART ONE, CHAPTER 8, #1

amino acids: basic organic compounds which are essential to the body's breakdown and absorption of foods. PART ONE, CHAPTER 11, #9

Bioplasma: a trademark name of a dietary supplement containing a combination of mineral salts, which the body uses. PART ONE, CHAPTER 4, #1

biotin: a vitamin which helps the body break down fats and is an aid in producing energy. PART ONE, CHAPTER 11, #2

bomb, like a: with considerable effectiveness or overwhelming success. PART ONE, CHAPTER 5, #2

brief (hold a brief for): support or defend. PART TWO, CHAPTER 5, #5

bulk fiber: the structural part of plants and plant products that are wholly or partially indigestible and when eaten help to move waste products through the intestines; roughage. PART ONE, CHAPTER 6, #2

catalytic: causing or accelerating a change without itself (the substance causing the change) being affected. PART ONE, CHAPTER 9, #3

choline: a vitamin important to the functioning of the nervous system, the liver and the buildup of immunities. PART ONE, CHAPTER 11, #3

cold-pressed: produced through extraction by low pressure without generating much heat and as a result retaining its nutritional value. PART ONE, CHAPTER 7, #1

cords: ropelike bands of tough, white tissue which connect the muscles to the bones in the body; tendons; sinews. PART ONE, CHAPTER 7, #3

Davis, Adelle: (1904–1973) prominent American nutritionist. PART ONE, CHAPTER 7, #4

DNA: a long, twisted protein found in all living cells primarily in the nucleus. It is the key to the development of cells, as it contains the hereditary "blueprint" needed to duplicate the cell as well as patterns for the production of specific other proteins needed by the body. PART ONE, CHAPTER 11, #11

dramatize: to repeat in action what has happened to one in experience. It is a replay now of something that happened in the past. PART TWO, CHAPTER 4, #2

empirical: derived from or guided by experience or experiment. PART TWO, CHAPTER 5, #6

endocrine system: the system of glands which produce one or more internal secretions that, introduced directly into the bloodstream, are carried to other parts of the body whose functions they regulate or control. PART ONE, CHAPTER 10, #1

euthanasia: the act or practice of painlessly putting to death an individual who is suffering from a terminal or incurable illness; "mercy killing." However, in the 1930s, a variation of euthanasia was used in Germany to rid the country of those considered burdens on society, including mentally defective people and alcoholics. Following on the heels of programs to sterilize people termed "unfit," euthanasia programs were employed in murdering over 200,000 mental patients from 1939 to 1945. These programs further expanded in the 1940s to include others considered "unworthy of life." PART ONE, CHAPTER 6, #3

exudation: the action of coming out gradually in drops, as sweat, through pores or small openings; oozing out. PART ONE, CHAPTER 2, #2

folic acid: a vitamin important in the formation of red blood cells. PART ONE, CHAPTER 11, #1

hypnotics: agents or drugs that produce sleep; sedatives. PART TWO, CHAPTER 5, #1

inositol: a B vitamin related to control of cholesterol level. PART ONE, CHAPTER 11, #5

iodine: a trace mineral that is vital for the production of growth hormones. It is extracted from seawater or seaweed, called kelp, which is rich in this mineral. PART ONE, CHAPTER 11, #8

ion: an electrically charged atom or group of atoms formed by the loss or gain of one or more electrons. A positive ion is created by electron loss, and a negative ion is created by electron gain. PART ONE, CHAPTER 8, #2

manganese: a mineral important to growth, bone formation, reproduction, muscle coordination and fat and carbohydrate metabolism. PART ONE, CHAPTER 11, #7

misemotion: anything that is unpleasant emotion such as antagonism, anger, fear, grief, apathy or a death feeling. PART TWO, CHAPTER 5, #4

Narconon: a social betterment organization and global network of drug rehabilitation and drug education centers, dedicated to restoring drug-free lives to drug dependent people through the use of L. Ron Hubbard's drug rehabilitation methods. PART ONE, CHAPTER 1, #3

objective: existing outside the mind as an actual object and not merely in the mind as an idea; real; about outward things not about the thoughts and feelings of the speaker. PART TWO, CHAPTER 2, #1

originations: a coined word meaning statements or remarks volunteered by a person concerning himself, his ideas, reactions or difficulties; communications originated by the person himself. PART TWO, CHAPTER 3, #1

overrun: the condition of continuing an action or a series of actions past the optimum point. PART TWO, CHAPTER 4, #1

PABA: an abbreviation for a vitamin called *para-amino-benzoic acid;* important in the metabolism of protein, blood cell formation, stimulation of intestinal bacteria to produce folic acid and utilization of pantothenic acid. PART ONE, CHAPTER 11, #6

pantothenic acid: one of the B vitamins, which is essential for cell growth. PART ONE, CHAPTER 11, #4

pharmacopeias: authoritative books containing lists and descriptions of drugs and medicinal products together with the standards established under law for their production, dispensation, use, etc. PART ONE, CHAPTER 9, #1

phenobarbital: a white crystalline powder used as a sedative and hypnotic. PART ONE, CHAPTER 1, #1

polyunsaturated: designates types of fat or oil that chemically contain fewer hydrogen atoms than they could hold; *poly—* many, *unsaturated—*not filled to capacity. These oils are obtained primarily from vegetables. Some of them are fats and oils required by the body that must be supplied through the diet because the body is not able to manufacture them. PART ONE, CHAPTER 7, #2

Program Case Supervisor: a properly certified person who is assigned the responsibility of overseeing the delivery of and ensuring the proper and exact application of all aspects of the Purification program to individuals. PART ONE, CHAPTER 5, #1

psychosomatic: *psycho* refers to mind and *somatic* refers to body; the term psychosomatic means the mind making the body ill or illnesses which have been created physically within the body by derangement of the mind. PART TWO, CHAPTER 5, #3

RNA: abbreviation for *ribonucleic acid;* one of the compounds found in all living cells; the substance that carries out DNA's instructions for protein production. PART ONE, CHAPTER 11, #12. *See also* **DNA.**

runs (something) out: causes some unwanted mental state or condition to erase. PART ONE, CHAPTER 9, #2

selenium: a trace mineral which helps to keep the body healthy, protect cells against oxidation and convert fat and protein to energy. PART ONE, CHAPTER 11, #10

somatics: physical pains or discomforts of any kind. The word *somatic* means, actually, bodily or physical. Because the word *pain* has in the past led to confusion between physical pain and mental pain, *somatic* is the term used to denote physical pain or discomfort. PART ONE, CHAPTER 9, #4

soporifics: drugs or medicines which induce sleep. PART TWO, CHAPTER 5, #2

trace minerals: those minerals which have been found essential to maintaining life, even though they are found in the body in very small, i.e., "trace" amounts. PART ONE, CHAPTER 10, #2

track: short for *time track,* the consecutive recording of mental image pictures which accumulates through a person's existence. APPENDIX A, #1

tranquilizers: drugs that have a sedative or calming effect without inducing sleep. PART ONE, CHAPTER 1, #2

wheat rust: a fungus which attacks wheat and produces reddish, brown or black marks resembling iron rust on the stems and leaves. The fungus penetrates the plant and forms a mass of filaments (the threadlike parts of a fungus) within the invaded tissue, and thus absorbs nourishment. PART ONE, CHAPTER 2, #1

INDEX

INDEX

FURTHER BOOKS AND LECTURES

BY L. RON HUBBARD

Further Books
and Lectures
by L. Ron Hubbard

THE BEST SOURCE OF INFORMATION on Dianetics and Scientology are the books and recorded lectures of L. Ron Hubbard. To guide you in learning more about Dianetics and Scientology, a selection of suggested books, lectures and videos is provided here.

The materials below have been laid out in a correct sequence for further reading and listening.

The wisdom of L. Ron Hubbard can be found in these materials. They are available to anyone who wants them. Many of these books are available in public bookstores and libraries; the rest can be obtained at any of the churches, missions or centers listed on page 217, or online at the addresses at the end of this section. Many of these books and lectures have been translated into a number of different languages.

Your Next Book

Purification: An Illustrated Answer to Drugs • This fully illustrated book describes the Purification program and exactly how it addresses the restimulative effects of drugs and toxins in the body. Included here in text and illustrations are the steps of the Purification program. This book fully illustrates how the program removes drugs and toxins that have been stored in the body, and how this purification restores the ability to think clearly, increases awareness and makes one far more able to improve as a spiritual being.

COMPANION MATERIALS TO *CLEAR BODY, CLEAR MIND*

All About Radiation • Written by L. Ron Hubbard and two well-known medical doctors, this book provides the facts surrounding the effect of radiation on the body and spirit and offers solutions to those harmful effects. An immediate sellout in bookstores when originally released, *All About Radiation* tells the truth about the little known and talked about subject of radiation, and introduces the Purification program as the technology to handle its cumulative effects. (See companion lecture series, *Radiation and Your Survival* where L. Ron Hubbard details the subject of radiation and its effects.)

> RADIATION AND YOUR SURVIVAL LECTURES • Shortly before the publication of *All About Radiation*, L. Ron Hubbard delivered a series of ten lectures where he fully detailed the subject of radiation and revealed some of the most significant discoveries ever made in this field. How does radiation affect an individual? What is nuclear fission? What effect do X-rays and gamma rays have on a person? What barrier must man surmount in order to survive? These questions and more are answered in this fascinating and vital series of lectures.

BASIC SCIENTOLOGY BOOKS

Scientology: The Fundamentals of Thought • L. Ron Hubbard regarded *The Fundamentals of Thought* as the first Scientology book. This work presents concise explanations of the most basic principles of Scientology: the cycle of action, the conditions of existence, the Affinity, Reality and Communication triangle and the parts of man—thetan (spirit), mind and body. It also includes a full chapter of processes anyone can apply to dramatically improve life.

The Problems of Work • Here, L. Ron Hubbard isolates the problems encountered on the job—whether on the assembly line or in the executive office and gives exact procedures for overcoming the exhaustion, stress, frustration and discontent of the workaday world. This book opens the door to efficiency and enthusiasm for work and life.

Scientology: A New Slant on Life • Thirty of L. Ron Hubbard's most popular essays reveal the broad application of Scientology to any area of life. Discover the exact anatomy of winning or losing, the root of marital success, helping children to be successful in their own lives, two rules for happy living, what problems are made of (and what resolves them), how knowledge affects one's certainty, the importance of honesty, the preservation of freedom and more. *Scientology: A New Slant on Life* contains both a discussion of the profound principles and concepts on which Scientology is based and remarkable practical techniques anyone can use to improve his life.

Scientology 0-8: The Book of Basics • A distillation of more than 40 million words of Scientology breakthroughs and technology, this book contains all the basics and principles of Scientology—the Scientology Axioms, the Aims of Scientology, the Code of a Scientologist and more than thirty scales and charts. The title means "Scientology, zero to infinity," the numeral 8 being the symbol for infinity standing upright. *Scientology 0-8* concisely provides all the central, fundamental data of life packed into one volume.

DIANETICS BOOKS, LECTURES & VIDEO

Dianetics: The Modern Science of Mental Health • Indisputably the most widely read and influential book on the human mind ever published. Hailed as a breakthrough "as revolutionary for humanity as the first caveman's discovery and utilization of fire," *Dianetics* has been a perennial bestseller for over five decades. Dianetics marks a turning point in man's knowledge and understanding of himself. In this book L. Ron Hubbard produces the first accurate description of the human mind, reveals the single source of all human irrationality, and provides a proven effective technology to clear away the barriers to a person's full mental potential. (See *Dianetics Lectures and Demonstrations* where

L. Ron Hubbard expands on his breakthrough discoveries and demonstrates Dianetics.)

HOW TO USE DIANETICS: A VISUAL GUIDEBOOK TO THE HUMAN MIND • This companion video to the book *Dianetics* visually describes the principles of the only workable technology of the mind and demonstrates how it is applied so you can put it into immediate application. In less than one hour this video shows you Dianetics procedure, step by step, so you can begin application of this life-changing technology.

DIANETICS LECTURES AND DEMONSTRATIONS • Following the release of *Dianetics: The Modern Science of Mental Health,* L. Ron Hubbard gave a special course in Dianetics to an audience in Oakland, California, eager to find out more about this breakthrough technology. In a series of four lectures, he expands on Dianetics principles and demonstrates Dianetics procedure.

FURTHER DIANETICS BOOKS & LECTURES

The Dynamics of Life • Written before *Dianetics: The Modern Science of Mental Health,* this book is the first formal record of L. Ron Hubbard's researches into the structure and functions of the human mind. This was the "original thesis" and includes the first description of Dianetics procedures and how they work. There are also case histories showing the unprecedented results of early Dianetics technology. Not surprisingly, when it was first circulated, Mr. Hubbard was deluged with requests for more information. This led him to write his landmark manual of the human mind, *Dianetics. The Dynamics of Life* offers a more concise view of how the mind works and how Dianetics can be used to alleviate man's suffering.

Dianetics: The Evolution of a Science • At a young age, L. Ron Hubbard became greatly intrigued by the mystery of man and his mind. *Dianetics: The Evolution of a Science* is the story of how he came to make the breakthroughs which solve this mystery. This book reveals how he was able to recognize and isolate an individual's true basic personality and details how painful or traumatic events in life can become fused with an individual's innermost self, causing fears, insecurities and psychosomatic ills. And it shows how, by first describing the full potential of the mind, he was able to discover these impediments. Because of his work, this potential is now attainable.

Science of Survival • Written the year following the explosive release of *Dianetics: The Modern Science of Mental Health,* L. Ron Hubbard urgently began writing this second book of Dianetics because so many more advances were being made. *Science of Survival* contains the first accurate prediction of human behavior. Here are the natural laws that predetermine how long and how well a person will survive. Understand these and you understand your friends, your associates, your family and even yourself. Organized around the Hubbard Chart of Human Evaluation, this book ensures your complete grasp of a subject as broad and essential as human behavior. You can place any person you know on this chart. At a glance you'll understand him or her better, and then predict what they'll do and how they'll respond in different situations. (See *The Science of Survival Lectures* where L. Ron Hubbard expands on his landmark book directly after its release.)

THE SCIENCE OF SURVIVAL LECTURES • In these two companion lectures to *Science of Survival,* L. Ron Hubbard covers his breakthrough discoveries from the book. With many examples and demonstrations, you'll learn to cut through the social veneer and see what really matters about people—their ethic level, how they handle truth, their courage level, ability to handle responsibility and more.

Self Analysis • This book will take you on the most interesting adventure of your life, the adventure of *you.* The barriers of life are really just shadows. *Self Analysis* shows you how to see through them and walk through them and be in the sun again. Use this simple volume of tests and techniques to increase abilities and raise your emotional tone level. Using this book for just 30 minutes a day can dramatically improve memory, reaction time, alertness, imagination and more. This is the adventure of Dianetics one can employ by himself right at home.

Child Dianetics • An indispensable guide for parents. Here are the basics of Dianetics applied to children including dozens of exercises, principles and simple procedures for handling childhood upsets and accidents and to help raise bright, happy children.

REFERENCE HANDBOOKS AND VIDEO

What Is Scientology? • All the information. All the facts. This book answers all questions about Scientology. The most comprehensive text ever assembled on the Scientology religion. This book covers its religious heritage, basic principles and practices, organizational structure, worldwide use and expansion, social betterment programs and much, much more. Contains hundreds of photographs, illustrations and charts. *What Is Scientology?* is the definitive reference for anyone who wants all the facts on the world's fastest growing religion.

The Scientology Handbook • A companion volume to *What Is Scientology?* this handbook covers the basic principles anyone needs to survive. Many people want to help others and would if only they knew what to do. This book fills that need. *The Scientology Handbook* provides miracle-working Scientology technology on how to preserve marriages, get delinquent children back in the fold, handle dissident elements in the society, get families out of the red, solve human conflict, handle illiteracy, resolve drug, alcohol and many other problems.

AN INTRODUCTION TO SCIENTOLOGY • This one-hour filmed interview, the only one ever granted by L. Ron Hubbard, explains how he made his discoveries and breakthroughs during his explorations of the mind, spirit and life. He discusses his bestseller, *Dianetics: The Modern Science of Mental Health,* and how Scientology came about. And he answers the most commonly asked questions: What is Scientology? Why is it a religion? What is the difference between the mind and the spirit? What is man's true purpose? How do people benefit from Scientology? And much more.

SCIENTOLOGY
CHURCHES
& MISSIONS

SCIENTOLOGY CHURCHES & MISSIONS

CHURCHES

UNITED STATES

ALBUQUERQUE
Church of Scientology
8106 Menaul Boulevard NE
Albuquerque, New Mexico 87110

ANN ARBOR
Church of Scientology
66 E. Michigan Avenue
Battle Creek, Michigan 49017

ATLANTA
Church of Scientology
1611 Mt. Vernon Road
Dunwoody, Georgia 30338

AUSTIN
Church of Scientology
2200 Guadalupe
Austin, Texas 78705

BOSTON
Church of Scientology
448 Beacon Street
Boston, Massachusetts 02115

BUFFALO
Church of Scientology
47 West Huron Street
Buffalo, New York 14202

CHICAGO
Church of Scientology
3011 North Lincoln Avenue
Chicago, Illinois 60657-4207

CINCINNATI
Church of Scientology
215 West 4th Street, 5th Floor
Cincinnati, Ohio 45202-2670

CLEARWATER
Church of Scientology
Flag Service Organization
210 S. Fort Harrison Avenue
Clearwater, Florida 33756

Foundation Church of Scientology
Flag Ship Service Organization
c/o *Freewinds* Relay Office
118 N. Fort Harrison Avenue
Clearwater, Florida 33755-4013

COLUMBUS
Church of Scientology
30 North High Street
Columbus, Ohio 43215

DALLAS
Church of Scientology
Celebrity Centre Dallas
1850 North Buckner Boulevard
Dallas, Texas 75228

DENVER
Church of Scientology
3385 South Bannock Street
Englewood, Colorado 80110

DETROIT
Church of Scientology
28000 Middlebelt Road
Farmington Hills, Michigan 48334

HONOLULU
Church of Scientology
1146 Bethel Street
Honolulu, Hawaii 96813

KANSAS CITY
Church of Scientology
2 East 39th Street
Kansas City, Missouri 64111

LAS VEGAS
Church of Scientology
846 East Sahara Avenue
Las Vegas, Nevada 89104

Church of Scientology
Celebrity Centre Las Vegas
4850 W. Flamingo Road, Ste. 10
Las Vegas, Nevada 89103

LONG ISLAND
Church of Scientology
99 Railroad Station Plaza
Hicksville, New York 11801-2850

LOS ANGELES AND VICINITY
Church of Scientology
of Los Angeles
4810 Sunset Boulevard
Los Angeles, California 90027

Church of Scientology
1451 Irvine Boulevard
Tustin, California 92680

Church of Scientology
1277 East Colorado Boulevard
Pasadena, California 91106

Church of Scientology
15643 Sherman Way
Van Nuys, California 91406

Church of Scientology
American Saint Hill
Organization
1413 L. Ron Hubbard Way
Los Angeles, California 90027

Church of Scientology
American Saint Hill Foundation
1413 L. Ron Hubbard Way
Los Angeles, California 90027

Church of Scientology
Advanced Organization
of Los Angeles
1306 L. Ron Hubbard Way
Los Angeles, California 90027

Church of Scientology
Celebrity Centre International
5930 Franklin Avenue
Hollywood, California 90028

LOS GATOS
Church of Scientology
2155 South Bascom Avenue,
Suite 120
Campbell, California 95008

MIAMI
Church of Scientology
120 Giralda Avenue
Coral Gables, Florida 33134

MINNEAPOLIS
Church of Scientology
Twin Cities
1011 Nicollet Mall
Minneapolis, Minnesota 55403

MOUNTAIN VIEW
Church of Scientology
117 Easy Street
Mountain View, California 94039

NASHVILLE
Church of Scientology
Celebrity Centre Nashville
1204 16th Avenue South
Nashville, Tennessee 37212

NEW HAVEN
Church of Scientology
909 Whalley Avenue
New Haven, Connecticut 06515-1728

NEW YORK CITY
Church of Scientology
227 West 46th Street
New York, New York 10036-1409

Church of Scientology
Celebrity Centre New York
65 East 82nd Street
New York, New York 10028

ORLANDO
Church of Scientology
1830 East Colonial Drive
Orlando, Florida 32803-4729

PHILADELPHIA
Church of Scientology
1315 Race Street
Philadelphia, Pennsylvania 19107

PHOENIX
Church of Scientology
2111 West University Drive
Mesa, Arizona 85201

PORTLAND
Church of Scientology
2636 NE Sandy Boulevard
Portland, Oregon 97232-2342

Church of Scientology
Celebrity Centre Portland
708 SW Salmon Street
Portland, Oregon 97205

SACRAMENTO
Church of Scientology
825 15th Street
Sacramento, California 95814-2096

SALT LAKE CITY
Church of Scientology
1931 South 1100 East
Salt Lake City, Utah 84106

SAN DIEGO
Church of Scientology
1330 4th Avenue
San Diego, California 92101

SAN FRANCISCO
Church of Scientology
83 McAllister Street
San Francisco, California 94102

SAN JOSE
Church of Scientology
80 East Rosemary Street
San Jose, California 95112

SANTA BARBARA
Church of Scientology
524 State Street
Santa Barbara, California 93101

SEATTLE
Church of Scientology
2226 3rd Avenue
Seattle, Washington 98121

ST. LOUIS
Church of Scientology
6901 Delmar Boulevard
University City, Missouri 63130

TAMPA
Church of Scientology
3617 Henderson Boulevard
Tampa, Florida 33609-4501

WASHINGTON, DC
Founding Church of Scientology
of Washington, DC
1701 20th Street NW
Washington, DC 20009

PUERTO RICO

HATO REY
Dianetics Center of Puerto Rico
272 JT Piñero Avenue
Hyde Park
San Juan, Puerto Rico 00918

CANADA

EDMONTON
Church of Scientology
10255 97th Street
Edmonton, Alberta
Canada T5J 0L9

KITCHENER
Church of Scientology
159–161 King Street West
Kitchener, Ontario
Canada N2G 1A6

MONTREAL
Church of Scientology
4489 Papineau Street
Montreal, Quebec
Canada H2H 1T7

OTTAWA
Church of Scientology
150 Rideau Street, 2nd Floor
Ottawa, Ontario
Canada K1N 5X6

QUEBEC
Church of Scientology
350 Bd Chareste Est
Quebec, Quebec
Canada G1K 3H5

TORONTO
Church of Scientology
696 Yonge Street, 2nd Floor
Toronto, Ontario
Canada M4Y 2A7

VANCOUVER
Church of Scientology
401 West Hastings Street
Vancouver, British Columbia
Canada V6B 1L5

WINNIPEG
Church of Scientology
315 Garry Street, Suite 210
Winnipeg, Manitoba
Canada R3B 2G7

UNITED KINGDOM

BIRMINGHAM
Church of Scientology
8 Ethel Street
Winston Churchill House
Birmingham, England B2 4BG

BRIGHTON
Church of Scientology
Third Floor, 79-83 North Street
Brighton, Sussex
England BN1 1ZA

EAST GRINSTEAD
Church of Scientology
Saint Hill Foundation
Saint Hill Manor
East Grinstead, West Sussex
England RH19 4JY

Advanced Organization
  Saint Hill
Saint Hill Manor
East Grinstead, West Sussex
England RH19 4JY

EDINBURGH
Hubbard Academy of Personal
  Independence
20 Southbridge
Edinburgh, Scotland EH1 1LL

LONDON
Church of Scientology
68 Tottenham Court Road
London, England W1P 0BB

Church of Scientology
Celebrity Centre London
42 Leinster Gardens
London, England W2 3AN

MANCHESTER
Church of Scientology
258 Deansgate
Manchester, England M3 4BG

PLYMOUTH
Church of Scientology
41 Ebrington Street
Plymouth, Devon
England PL4 9AA

SUNDERLAND
Church of Scientology
51 Fawcett Street
Sunderland, Tyne and Wear
England SR1 1RS

EUROPE

AUSTRIA
VIENNA
Church of Scientology
Schottenfeldgasse 13/15
1070 Vienna, Austria

Church of Scientology
Celebrity Centre Vienna
Senefeldergasse 11/5
1100 Vienna, Austria

BELGIUM
BRUSSELS
Church of Scientology
rue General MacArthur, 9
1180 Brussels, Belgium

DENMARK
AARHUS
Church of Scientology
Vester Alle 26
8000 Aarhus C, Denmark

COPENHAGEN
Church of Scientology
Store Kongensgade 55
1264 Copenhagen K, Denmark

Church of Scientology of Denmark
Gammel Kongevej 3–5, 1
1610 Copenhagen V, Denmark

Church of Scientology
Advanced Organization
   Saint Hill for Europe and Africa
Jernbanegade 6
1608 Copenhagen V, Denmark

FRANCE
ANGERS
Church of Scientology
28B, avenue Mendès
49240 Avrille, France

CLERMONT-FERRAND
Church of Scientology
6, rue Dulaure
63000 Clermont-Ferrand
France

LYON
Church of Scientology
3, place des Capucins
69001 Lyon, France

PARIS
Church of Scientology
7, rue Jules César
75012 Paris, France

Church of Scientology
Celebrity Centre Paris
69, rue Legendre
75017 Paris, France

SAINT-ÉTIENNE
Church of Scientology
24, rue Marengo
42000 Saint-Étienne, France

GERMANY
BERLIN
Church of Scientology
Sponholzstraße 51–52
12159 Berlin 41
Germany

DÜSSELDORF

Church of Scientology
Friedrichstraße 28B
40217 Düsseldorf, Germany

Church of Scientology
Celebrity Centre Düsseldorf
Rheinland e. V.
Luisenstraße 23
40215 Düsseldorf, Germany

FRANKFURT

Church of Scientology
Kaiserstraße 49
60329 Frankfurt 70
Germany

HAMBURG

Church of Scientology
Domstraße 9
20095 Hamburg, Germany

Church of Scientology
Brennerstraße 12
20099 Hamburg, Germany

HANOVER

Church of Scientology
Odeonstraße 17
30159 Hanover, Germany

MUNICH

Church of Scientology
Beichstraße 12
80802 Munich 40
Germany

STUTTGART

Church of Scientology
Hohenheimerstraße 9
70184 Stuttgart, Germany

HUNGARY

BUDAPEST

Church of Scientology
1399 Budapest
1073 Erzsébet krt. 5. I. em.
Pf. 701/215. Hungary

ISRAEL

TEL AVIV

Scientology Center
12 Shontzino Street
PO Box 57478
61573 Tel Aviv, Israel

ITALY

BRESCIA

Church of Scientology
Via Fratelli Bronzetti, 20
25125 Brescia, Italy

CATANIA

Church of Scientology
Via Garibaldi, 9
95121 Catania, Italy

MILAN

Church of Scientology
Via Lepontina, 4
20159 Milan, Italy

MONZA

Church of Scientology
Via Ghilini, 4
20052 Monza (MI), Italy

NOVARA

Church of Scientology
Corso Milano, 28
28100 Novara, Italy

NUORO

Church of Scientology
Via Lamarmora, 102
08100 Nuoro, Italy

PADUA

Church of Scientology
Via Ugo Foscolo, 5
35131 Padua, Italy

PORDENONE

Church of Scientology
Via Dogana, 19
Zona Fiera
33170 Pordenone, Italy

ROME
Church of Scientology
Via del Caravita, 5
00186 Rome, Italy

TURIN
Church of Scientology
Via Bersezio, 7
10152 Turin, Italy

VERONA
Church of Scientology
Corso Milano, 84
37138 Verona, Italy

NETHERLANDS

AMSTERDAM
Church of Scientology
Nieuwezijds Voorburgwal
116–118 1012 SH
Amsterdam, Netherlands

NORWAY

OSLO
Church of Scientology
Storgata 17
0184 Oslo, Norway

PORTUGAL

LISBON
Church of Scientology
Rua dos Correiros N 205,
  3° Andar
1100 Lisbon, Portugal

RUSSIA

MOSCOW
Hubbard Humanitarian Center
Ul. Boris Galushkina 19A
129301 Moscow, Russia

SPAIN

BARCELONA
Dianetics Civil Association
Pasaje Domingo, 11–13 Bahos
08007 Barcelona, Spain

MADRID
Dianetics Civil Association
Villa Maria
C/ Montera 20, Piso 1° dcha.
28013 Madrid, Spain

SWEDEN

GÖTEBORG
Church of Scientology
Värmlandsgatan 16, 1 tr.
413 28 Göteborg, Sweden

MALMÖ
Church of Scientology
Porslinsgatan 3
211 32 Malmö, Sweden

STOCKHOLM
Church of Scientology
Götgatan 105
116 62 Stockholm, Sweden

SWITZERLAND

BASEL
Church of Scientology
Herrengrabenweg 56
4054 Basel, Switzerland

BERN
Church of Scientology
Muhlemattstrasse 31
Postfach 384
3000 Bern 14, Switzerland

GENEVA
Church of Scientology
12, rue des Acacias
1227 Carouge
Geneva, Switzerland

LAUSANNE
Church of Scientology
10, rue de la Madeleine
1003 Lausanne, Switzerland

ZURICH
Church of Scientology
Freilagerstrasse 11
8047 Zurich, Switzerland

AUSTRALIA

ADELAIDE

Church of Scientology
24–28 Waymouth Street
Adelaide, South Australia
Australia 5000

BRISBANE

Church of Scientology
106 Edward Street, 2nd Floor
Brisbane, Queensland
Australia 4000

CANBERRA

Church of Scientology
43–45 East Row
Canberra City, ACT
Australia 2601

MELBOURNE

Church of Scientology
42–44 Russell Street
Melbourne, Victoria
Australia 3000

PERTH

Church of Scientology
108 Murray Street, 1st Floor
Perth, Western Australia
Australia 6000

SYDNEY

Church of Scientology
201 Castlereagh Street
Sydney, New South Wales
Australia 2000

Church of Scientology
Advanced Organization
  Saint Hill Australia,
  New Zealand and Oceania
19–37 Greek Street
Glebe, New South Wales
Australia 2037

JAPAN

TOKYO

Scientology Tokyo
2-11-7, Kita-otsuka
Toshima-ku
Tokyo, Japan 170-0004

NEW ZEALAND

AUCKLAND

Church of Scientology
532 Ellerslie/Panmure Highway
Panmure, Auckland, New Zealand

AFRICA

BULAWAYO

Church of Scientology
Southampton House, Suite 202
Main Street and 9th Avenue
Bulawayo, Zimbabwe

CAPE TOWN

Church of Scientology
Ground Floor, Dorlane House
39 Roeland Street
Cape Town 8001, South Africa

DURBAN

Church of Scientology
20 Buckingham Terrace
Westville, Durban 3630
South Africa

HARARE

Church of Scientology
404-409 Pockets Building
50 Jason Moyo Avenue
Harare, Zimbabwe

JOHANNESBURG

Church of Scientology
4th Floor, Budget House
130 Main Street
Johannesburg 2001
South Africa

Church of Scientology
No. 108 1st Floor,
  Bordeaux Centre
Gordon Road, Corner Jan
  Smuts Avenue
Blairgowrie, Randburg 2125
South Africa

PORT ELIZABETH

Church of Scientology
2 St. Christopher's
27 Westbourne Road Central
Port Elizabeth 6001
South Africa

PRETORIA

Church of Scientology
307 Ancore Building
Corner Jeppe and Esselen Streets
Sunnyside, Pretoria 0002
South Africa

LATIN AMERICA

ARGENTINA

BUENOS AIRES

Dianetics Association of Argentina
2162 Bartolomé Mitre
Capital Federal
Buenos Aires 1039, Argentina

COLOMBIA

BOGOTÁ

Dianetics Cultural Center
Carrera 30 #91–96
Bogotá, Colombia

MEXICO

GUADALAJARA

Dianetics Cultural
  Organization, A.C.
Avenida de la Paz 2787
Fracc. Arcos Sur
Sector Juárez, Guadalajara, Jalisco
CP 44500, Mexico

MEXICO CITY

Dianetics Cultural
  Association, A.C.
Belisario Domínguez #17-1
Villa Coyoacán
Colonia Coyoacán
CP 04000, Mexico, D.F.

Institute of Applied
  Philosophy, A.C.
Municipio Libre No. 40
Esq. Mira Flores
Colonia Portales
Mexico, D.F.

Latin American Cultural
  Center, A.C.
Rio Amazonas 11
Colonia Cuahutemoc
CP 06500, Mexico, D.F.

Dianetics Technological
  Institute, A.C.
Avenida Chapultepec 540, 6° Piso
Colonia Roma, Metro
Chapultepec
CP 06700, Mexico, D.F.

Dianetics Development
  Organization, A.C.
San Luis Potosi 196 #3er Piso
Esq. Medellin
Colonia Roma
CP 06700, Mexico, D.F.

Dianetics Cultural
  Organization, A.C.
Calle Monterrey #402
Colonia Narvarte
CP 03020, Mexico, D.F.

VENEZUELA

CARACAS

Dianetics Cultural
  Organization, A.C.
Calle Caciquiare
Entre Yumare y Atures
Quinta Shangai
Urbanización El Marquez
Caracas, Venezuela

VALENCIA

Dianetics Cultural
  Association, A.C.
Ave. Bolívar Norte
Urbanización el Viñedo
Edificio "Mi Refugio" #141–45
A 30 Metros de Ave,
Monseñor Adams
Valencia, Edo Carabobo, Venezuela

MISSIONS

INTERNATIONAL OFFICE

Scientology Missions International
6331 Hollywood Boulevard
  Suite 501
Los Angeles, California 90028-6314

UNITED STATES

Scientology Missions International
Western United States Office
1308 L. Ron Hubbard Way
Los Angeles, California 90027

Scientology Missions International
Eastern United States Office
349 W. 48th Street
New York, New York 10036

Scientology Missions International
Flag Land Base Office
210 S. Fort Harrison Avenue
Clearwater, Florida 33756

MISSIONS AND DIANETICS CENTERS

ALASKA

Church of Scientology
Mission of Anchorage
1300 East 68th Avenue
  Suite 112
Anchorage, Alaska 99508

CALIFORNIA

Church of Scientology
Mission of Antelope Valley
5308 W. M–4
Quartz Hill, California 93536

Church of Scientology
Mission of Auburn
4035 Grass Valley Hwy J
Auburn, California 95602

Church of Scientology
Mission of Berkeley (Bay Cities)
2975 Treat Boulevard, Suite D-4
Concord, California 94518

Church of Scientology
Mission of Beverly Hills
9885 Charleville Boulevard
Beverly Hills, California 90212

Church of Scientology
Mission of Brand Boulevard
222 1/2 N. Brand Blvd.
Glendale, California 91205–32160

Church of Scientology
Mission of Buenaventura
180 North Ashwood Avenue
Ventura, California 93003

Church of Scientology
Mission of Burbank
6623 Irvine Avenue
North Hollywood, California 91607

Church of Scientology
Mission of Capitol
9915 Fair Oaks Boulevard
  Suite A
Fair Oaks, California 95628

Church of Scientology
Mission of Costa Mesa
4706 E. Bond Avenue
Orange, California 92869

Church of Scientology
Mission of the Diablo Valley
801-B "A" Street
Antioch, California 94509

Church of Scientology
Mission of Escondido
326 South Kalmia Street
Escondido, California 92025

Church of Scientology
Mission of the Foothills
2254 Honolulu Avenue
Montrose, California 91020

Church of Scientology
Mission of Inglewood
133 N. Prairie Avenue
Inglewood, California 90301

Church of Scientology
Mission of Los Angeles (Russian)
13059 Oxnard Street, Apt. #208
Van Nuys, California 91401

Church of Scientology
Mission of Malibu
c/o 222 1/2 N. Brand Blvd.
Glendale, California 91203-2610

Church of Scientology
Mission of Los Angeles
5408 Carpenter Avenue #204
North Hollywood, California 91607

Church of Scientology
Mission of Marin
1930 4th Street
San Rafael, California 94901

Church of Scientology
Mission of Montebello
(Spanish LA)
17904 Hurley Street
La Puente, California 91744

Church of Scientology
Mission of Newport Beach
3905 Channel Place
Newport Beach, California 92663

Church of Scientology
Mission of Orange
415 N. Tustin Avenue
Orange, California 92867

Church of Scientology
Mission of Palo Alto
3505 El Camino Real
Palo Alto, California 94306

Church of Scientology
Mission of Redondo Beach
3620 Pacific Coast Highway
Redondo Beach, California 90505

Church of Scientology
Mission of Redwood City
617 Veterans Boulevard, #205
Redwood City, California 94063

Church of Scientology
Mission of River Park
1010 Hurley Way, Suite 505
Sacramento, California 95825

Church of Scientology
Mission of San Bernardino
5 East Citrus Avenue, Suite 105
Redlands, California 92373

Church of Scientology
Mission of San Francisco
701 Sutter Street, 3rd Floor
San Francisco, California 94109

Church of Scientology
Mission of San Jose
826 North Winchester Boulevard
  Suite 1
San Jose, California 95128

Church of Scientology
Mission of Santa Clara Valley
3596 Calico Avenue
San Jose, California 95124

Church of Scientology
Mission of Santa Monica
1337 Ocean Avenue #C
Santa Monica, California 90410

Church of Scientology
Mission of Santa Rosa
850 2nd Street, Suite F
Santa Rosa, California 95404

Church of Scientology
Mission of Sherman Oaks
13517 Ventura Boulevard, #8
Sherman Oaks, California 91423

Church of Scientology
Mission of SoMa
966 Mission Street
San Francisco, California 94102

Church of Scientology
Mission of Temecula
40935 Country Center Drive,
Temecula, California 92591

Church of Scientology
Mission of Thousand Oaks
c/o 21010 Devonshire Street
Chatsworth, California 91311

Church of Scientology
Mission of Torrance
3620 Pacific Coast Highway
Torrance, California 90505

Church of Scientology
Mission of West Valley
21010 Devonshire Street
Chatsworth, California 91311

Church of Scientology
Mission of Westwood
3109 Carter Avenue
Marina Del Rey, California 90292

COLORADO

Church of Scientology
Mission of Alamosa
511 Main Street, Suite #6
Alamosa, Colorado 81101

Church of Scientology
Mission of Boulder
1021 Pearl Street
Boulder, Colorado 80302

Church of Scientology
Mission of Roaring Fork
827 Bennett Avenue
Glenwood Springs, Colorado 81601

DELAWARE

Church of Scientology
Mission of Collingswood
PO Box 730
Claymont, Delaware 19703-0730

FLORIDA

Church of Scientology
Mission of Belleair
2907 West Bay Drive
Belleair Bluffs, Florida 33770

Church of Scientology
Mission of Clearwater
100 North Belcher Road
Clearwater, Florida 33765

Church of Scientology
Mission of Fort Lauderdale
660 South Federal Highway
   Suite 200
Pompano Beach, Florida 33062

Church of Scientology
Mission of Palm Harbor
5 Birdie Lane
Palm Harbor, Florida 34683

Church of Scientology
Mission of Palm Harbor
5 Birdie Lane
Palm Harbor, Florida 34683

Church of Scientology
Mission of Sarasota
6576 Superior Avenue
Sarasota, Florida 34231

HAWAII

Church of Scientology
Mission of Honolulu
6172 May Way
Honolulu, Hawaii 96821

ILLINOIS

Church of Scientology
Mission of Champaign-Urbana
312 West John Street
Champaign, Illinois 61820

Church of Scientology
Mission of Chicago
6107 B. North NW Highway
Chicago, Illinois 60631

Church of Scientology
Mission of Peoria
2020 North Wisconsin
Peoria, Illinois 61603

KANSAS

Church of Scientology
Mission of Wichita
3705 East Douglas
Wichita, Kansas 67218

LOUISIANA

Church of Scientology
Mission of Baton Rouge
9432 Common Street
Baton Rouge, Louisiana 70806

Church of Scientology
Mission of Lafayette
102 Huggins Road
Lafayette, Louisiana 70506

MAINE

Church of Scientology
Mission of Brunswick
2 Lincoln Street
Brunswick, Maine 04011

MASSACHUSETTS

Church of Scientology
Mission of Boston
c/o 142 Primrose Street
Haverhill, Massachusetts 01830

Church of Scientology
Mission of Merrimack Valley
142 Primrose Street
Haverhill, Massachusetts 01830

Church of Scientology
Mission of Watertown
313 Common Street #2
Watertown, Massachusetts 02472

MICHIGAN

Church of Scientology
Mission of Genesee County
423 North Saginaw
Holly, Michigan 48442

Church of Scientology
Mission of Rochester Hills
3650 Galloway Ct. #2908
Rochester Hills, Michigan 48309

NEBRASKA

Church of Scientology
Mission of Omaha
843 Hidden Hills Drive
Bellevue, Nebraska 68005

NEVADA

Church of Scientology
Mission of Las Vegas
2923 Schaffer Circle
Las Vegas, Nevada 89121

Church of Scientology
Mission of Sierra Nevada
1539 Vassar Street, Suite 201
Reno, Nevada 89502-2745

Church of Scientology
Mission of Vegas Valley
7545 Bermuda Road
Las Vegas, Nevada 89123

NEW HAMPSHIRE

Church of Scientology
Mission of Greater Concord
Suite 3C-4 Bicentennial Square
Concord, New Hampshire 03301

NEW JERSEY

Church of Scientology
Mission of Elizabeth
433 North Broad Street
Elizabeth, New Jersey 07208

Church of Scientology
Mission of New Jersey
1029 Teaneck Road
Teaneck, New Jersey 07666

NEW YORK

Church of Scientology
Mission of Middletown
21 Mill Street
Liberty, New York 12754

Church of Scientology
Mission of Queens
56-03 214th Street
Bayside, New York 11364

Church of Scientology
Mission of Rochester
4178 Holley Byron Road
Holley, New York 14470

Church of Scientology
Mission of Westchester
11 Holland Avenue, White Plains
Westchester, New York 10603

PENNSYLVANIA

Church of Scientology
Mission of Pittsburgh
220 Nazareth Drive
Belle Vernon
Pennsylvania 15012

SOUTH CAROLINA

Church of Scientology
Mission of Charleston
PO Box 606
Santee, South Carolina 29142

TENNESSEE

Church of Scientology
Mission of Memphis
1440 Central Avenue
Memphis, Tennessee 38104

TEXAS

Church of Scientology
Mission of El Paso
1120 North El Paso Street
El Paso, Texas 79902

Church of Scientology
Mission of Harlingen
4301 W. Business 83
Harlingen, Texas 78552

Church of Scientology
Mission of Houston
2727 Fondren, Suite 1-A
Houston, Texas 77063

Church of Scientology
Mission of San Antonio
5119 Fort Clark Drive
Austin, Texas 78745

VIRGINIA

Church of Scientology
Mission of Piedmont
17203 James Madison Hwy
Gordonsville, Virginia 22942

WASHINGTON

Church of Scientology
Mission of Bellevue
15424 Bellevue-Redmond Road
Redmond, Washington 98052

Church of Scientology
Mission of Bellingham
722 N. State Street
Bellingham, Washington 98225

Church of Scientology
Mission of Burien
15216 2nd Avenue SW
Seattle, Washington 98166

Church of Scientology
Mission of Seattle
1234 NE 145th Street
Seattle, Washington 98155

Dianetics Center
Mission of Spokane
1810 North Ruby
Spokane, Washington 99207

WISCONSIN

Church of Scientology
Mission of Milwaukee
710 East Silver Spring Drive
   Suite E
Whitefish Bay, Wisconsin 53217

AFRICA

Scientology Missions
  International
African Office
6th Floor, Budget House
130 Main Street
Johannesburg 2001, South Africa

MISSIONS AND DIANETICS CENTERS

Church of Scientology
Mission of Kinshasa
BP 1444
7, rue de Fele
Kinshasa/Limete, Zaire

Church of Scientology
Mission of Lagos
16 Moor Road
Off University Road, Yaba
Lagos, Nigeria
West Africa

Church of Scientology
Mission of Norwood
18 Trilby Street
Oaklands, Johannesburg 2192
Republic of South Africa

Church of Scientology
Mission of Soweto
PO Box 890019
Lyndhurst
Republic of South Africa

AUSTRALIA, NEW ZEALAND AND OCEANIA

Scientology Missions
  International
Australian, New Zealand
  and Oceanian Office
201 Castlereagh Street, 3rd Floor
Sydney, New South Wales
Australia 2000

MISSIONS AND DIANETICS CENTERS

AUSTRALIA

Church of Scientology
Mission of Inner West Sydney
4 Wangal Place
Five Dock, New South Wales
Australia 2046

Church of Scientology
Mission of Melbourne
55 Glenferrie Road
Malvern, Victoria
Australia 3144

NEW ZEALAND

Church of Scientology
Mission of Christchurch
PO Box 1843
Christchurch
New Zealand

CANADA

Scientology Missions
  International
Canadian Office
696 Yonge Street
Toronto, Ontario
Canada M4Y 2A7

MISSIONS AND DIANETICS CENTERS

Church of Scientology
Mission of Beauce
3020 127. #7
Ville de St-Georges
Beauce, Quebec
Canada G5Y 6K9

Church of Scientology
Mission of Calgary
Box 22
Site 2 RR1
Millerville, Alberta
Canada T0L 1K0

Church of Scientology
Mission of Halifax
6100 Young Street #300
Halifax, Nova Scotia
Canada B3K 2A4

Church of Scientology
Mission of Montreal
1690 A, avenue de l'Église
Montreal, Quebec
Canada H4E 1G5

Church of Scientology
Mission of Toronto
2007 Danforth Avenue
Toronto, Ontario
Canada M4C 1J7

Church of Scientology
Mission of Vancouver
2860 West 4th Avenue
Vancouver, British Columbia
Canada V6K 1R2

Church of Scientology
Chinese Mission of Vancouver
609–6651 Minoru Blvd.
Richmond, British Columbia
Canada V6Y 1Z2

Church of Scientology
Mission of Victoria
1319 Douglas Street
Victoria, British Columbia
Canada V8W 2E9

EUROPE

Scientology Missions
  International
European Office
Store Kongensgade 55
1264 Copenhagen K
Denmark

MISSIONS AND DIANETICS CENTERS

ALBANIA

Church of Scientology
Mission of Tirana
Rr "Bardhyl" PL. 18 shk: 2
AP: 3
Tirana, Albania

AUSTRIA

Scientology Mission Salzburg
Rupertgasse 21
5020 Salzburg, Austria

Scientology Mission Wolfsberg
Am Weiher 10
9400 Wolfsberg, Austria

CROATIA

Church of Scientology
Mission of Zagreb
Tkalciceva 76
10000 Zagreb
Croatia

CZECH REPUBLIC

Dianetics Center
Jindrisska 7
110 00 Prague 10
Czech Republic

DENMARK

Church of Scientology
Mission of Aalborg
Boulevarden 39 st.
9000 Aalborg, Denmark

Church of Scientology
Mission of Copenhagen City
Rathsacksvej 1, 4th floor
1862 Frederiksberg C
Denmark

Church of Scientology
Mission of Fyn
Ove Gjeddes Vej. 27
5220 Odense
Denmark

Church of Scientology
Mission of Lyngby
Sorgenfrivej 3
2800 Lyngby, Denmark

Church of Scientology
Mission of Silkeborg
Virklundvej 5, Virklund
8600 Silkeborg, Denmark

FINLAND

Church of Scientology
Mission of Helsinki
Peltolantie 2 B
01300 Vantaa, Finland

Church of Scientology
Dianetiikka-keskus
Hämeenkatu 11 D
15110 Lahti, Finland

FRANCE

Church of Scientology
Mission of Bordeaux
41, rue de Cheverus
33000 Bordeaux, France

Church of Scientology
Mission of Marseille
2, rue Devilliers
13005 Marseille, France

Church of Scientology
Mission of Nice
28, rue Gioffredo
06000 Nice, France

Church of Scientology
Mission of Toulouse
9, rue Edmond de Planet
31000 Toulouse, France

GERMANY

Scientology Mission Augsburg
Frauentorstr. 40
86152 Augsburg, Germany

Scientology Mission Bremen e.V.
Stolzenauer Str. 36
28207 Bremen, Germany

Dianetik Göppingen e.V.
Scientology Mission
Geislingerstraße 21
73033 Göppingen, Germany

Scientology Heilbronn
Mission der Scientology
  Kirche e.V.
Am Wollhaus 8
74072 Heilbronn, Germany

Mission der Scientology Kirche
Karlstraße 46
76133 Karlsruhe, Germany

Scientology Mission Pasing
Landsbergstraße 416
81241 Munich, Germany

Scientology Kirche Bayern e.V.
Gemeinde Nuremberg
Färberstraße 5
90402 Nuremberg, Germany

Scientology Mission e.V.
Heinestraße 9
72762 Reutlingen, Germany

Scientology Mission Ulm e.V.
Eythstraße 2
89075 Ulm, Germany

GREECE

Greek Dianetics and
  Scientology Centre
Patision 200
11256 Athens, Greece

ITALY

Scientology Missions
  International
Italian Office
Via Cadorna, 61
20090 Vimodrone (MI), Italy

MISSIONS AND
DIANETICS CENTERS
Church of Scientology
Mission of Aosta
Corso Battaglione, 13/B
11100 Aosta, Italy

Church of Scientology
Mission of Assemini
Via Sardegna, 117
09032 Assemini (CA), Cagliari

Church of Scientology
Mission of Asti
Corso Alfieri, 51
14100 Asti, Italy

Church of Scientology
Mission of Avellino
Via Fratelli Bisogno, 5
83100 Avellino, Italy

Church of Scientology
Mission of Barletta
Via Cialdini, 67/B
70051 Barletta (BA), Italy

Church of Scientology
Mission of Bergamo
Via Roma, 85
24020 Gorle (BG), Italy

Church of Scientology
Mission of Bologna
Via delle Fragole, 14
40127 Bologna, Italy

Church of Scientology
Mission of Bolzano
Via Al Boschetto, 7
39100 Bolzano, Italy

Church of Scientology
Mission of Cagliari
Via Sonnino, 177
09127 Cagliari, Italy

Church of Scientology
Mission of Cantù
Via G. da Fossano, 40
22063 Cantù (CO), Italy

Church of Scientology
Mission of Carpi
Via Trento Trieste, 59
41012 Carpi (MO), Italy

Church of Scientology
Mission of Castelfranco
Piazza Serenissima, 40
31033 Castelfranco Veneto (TV), Italy

Church of Scientology
Mission of Como
Via Torno, 12
22100 Como, Italy

Church of Scientology
Mission of Conegliano
Via Manin, 9
31015 Conegliano (TV), Italy

Church of Scientology
Mission of Cosenza
Via Duca degli Abruzzi, 6
87100 Cosenza, Italy

Church of Scientology
Mission of Franciacorta
Via de Gasperi, 6
25040 Nigoline
   di Cortefranca (BS)
Italy

Church of Scientology
Mission of Lecco
Via Mascari, 78
23900 Lecco, Italy

Church of Scientology
Mission of Lucca
Viale G. Puccini, 425/B
55100 Lucca, Italy

Church of Scientology
Mission of Macerata
Via Moretti, 1
62010 Piediripa (MC), Italy

Church of Scientology
Mission of Mantova
Via Alberto Mario, 21
46100 Mantova, Italy

Church of Scientology
Mission of Merate
Via Paolo Arlati (Ang. Via Roma)
23807 Merate (LC), Italy

Church of Scientology
Mission of Milano
Via Vannucci, 13
20135 Milano, Italy

Church of Scientology
Mission of Modena
Via Giardini, 468/C
41100 Modena, Italy

Church of Scientology
Mission of Olbia
Via Gabriele D'Annunzio, 13
c/o Martini
07026 Olbia (SS), Italy

Church of Scientology
Mission of Palermo
Via Mariano Stabile, 139
90100 Palermo, Italy

Church of Scientology
Mission of Ragusa
Via Caporale degli Zuavi, 67
97019 Vittoria (RG), Italy

Church of Scientology
Mission of Romano (Clusone)
Via G. Rubini, 12
24045 Romano
  di Lombardia (BG), Italy

Church of Scientology
Mission of Roncadelle
Vicolo del Mattino, 3
25030 Roncadelle (BS), Italy

Church of Scientology
Mission of Treviglio
Via Bicetti, 8A
24047 Treviglio (BG), Italy

Church of Scientology
Mission of Trieste
Via Gatteri, 28
34129 Trieste, Italy

Church of Scientology
Mission of Vicenza Centro
Via Contra Manin, 20
36100 Vicenza, Italy

MACEDONIA

Hubbard Center for Dianetics
  and Scientology
Bul. Partizanski Odredi 21/1
Deloven Kompleks "Porta
  Bunjakovec"
Mezzanine A 3/2
1000 Skopje
Republic of Macedonia

ROMANIA

Dianetics Center of Nagyvarad
3700 Oradea
Str. Progresului nr. 40
BL B-19-20. ap. 5
Romania

Dianetics Center of
  Székelyudvarhely
4150 Odorheiu Secuiesc
Str. M. Sadoveanu 13
CP: 28
Romania

SLOVENIA

Dianetics Centre of Koper
Za Gradom, 21
6000 Koper
Slovenia

SPAIN

Centro de Eficiencia
  Personal Dianética
C/ Hermanos Rivas, 22-1-1A
46018 Valencia, Spain

Centro de Mejoramiento
  Personal
C/ Viera y Clavijo, 33-2 Planta
35002 Las Palmas de Gran Canaria
Spain

Centro de Mejoramiento
  Personal
Urbanización Los Mirtos, 65
41020 Sevilla, Spain

Centro de Mejoramiento
   Personal de Cercedilla
Cambrils, 19
28034 Madrid, Spain

Misión de la Moraleja
Cuesta Blanca, 213
28100 Madrid, Spain

SWEDEN

Dianetik Huset
Finnbodavägen 2, 4th
13131 Nacka, Sweden

SWITZERLAND

Church of Scientology
Mission of Lugano
Via Campagna, 30A
6982 Serocca D'Agno
Switzerland

Dianetik and Scientology
   Luzern Mission
Zentrum für
   Angewandte Philosophie
Sentimattstrasse 7
6011 Luzern, Switzerland

Mission der Scientology Kirche
Regensbergstrasse 89
8050 Zürich, Switzerland

CENTRAL EUROPE

Scientology Missions
   International
Central European Office
1438 Budapest
Pf. 351
Hungary

MISSIONS AND DIANETICS CENTERS

Church of Scientology
Mission of Baja
6500 Baja
Galamb u. 13.
Hungary

Church of Scientology
Mission of Belváros
1052 Budapest
Károly krt. 4. III/10.
Hungary

Church of Scientology
Mission of Bonyhád
7150 Bonyhád
Bartók Béla u. 56/A
Hungary

Church of Scientology
Mission of Debrecen
4031 Debrecen
Derék u. 181. 4/12
Hungary

Church of Scientology
Mission of Dunaújváros
2404 Dunaújváros
Pf. 435
Hungary

Church of Scientology
Mission of Eger
3300 Eger
Pf. 215
Hungary

Church of Scientology
Mission of Esztergom
2500 Esztergom
Budapesti út 30.
Hungary

Church of Scientology
Mission of Győr
9026 Győr
Dózsa György rakpart 1/4.
Hungary

Church of Scientology
Mission of Kalocsa
6300 Kalocsa
Alkotás u. 20. II/7
Hungary

Church of Scientology
Mission of Kaposvár
7400 Kaposvár
Ûrhajós u. 38. 1/1
Hungary

Church of Scientology
Mission of Kazincbarcika
3700 Kazincbarcika
Ságvári tér 3.
Hungary

Church of Scientology
Mission of Keszthely
8360 Keszthely
Sopron u. 41.
Hungary

Church of Scientology
Mission of Kiskunfélegyháza
6101 Kiskunfélegyháza
Pf. 23
Hungary

Church of Scientology
Mission of Mezőkövesd
3400 Mezőkövesd
Dr. Lukács Gáspár u. 5.
Hungary

Church of Scientology
Mission of Miskolc
3530 Miskolc
Széchenyi u. 34. I. em.
Hungary

Church of Scientology
Mission of Nyíregyháza
4400 Nyíregyháza
Vasvári Pál út 14.
Hungary

Church of Scientology
Mission of Ózd
3600 Ózd
Sárlitelep
Hungary

Church of Scientology
Mission of Paks
7030 Paks
Kodály Zoltán u. 30
Pf. 10
Hungary

Church of Scientology
Mission of Pécs
7621 Pécs
Király u. 8.
7602 Pécs 2
Pf. 41
Hungary

Church of Scientology
Mission of Sopron
9401 Sopron
Pf. 111
Hungary

Church of Scientology
Mission of Százhalombatta
2440 Százhalombatta
Pf. 69
Hungary

Church of Scientology
Mission of Szeged
6722 Szeged
Pf. 1258
Hungary

Church of Scientology
Mission of Székesfehérvár
8001 Székesfehérvár
Pf. 176
Hungary

Church of Scientology
Mission of Szekszárd
7100 Szekszárd
Pf. 165
Hungary

Church of Scientology
Mission of Tatabánya
2800 Tatabánya
Pf. 1372
Hungary

Church of Scientology
Mission of Tiszaújváros
3580 Tiszaújváros
Teleki Blanka u. 2.
Hungary

Church of Scientology
Mission of Veszprém
8200 Veszprém
Völgyhíd tér 3.
Hungary

COMMONWEALTH OF INDEPENDENT STATES

Scientology Missions
  International
CIS Office
Hubbard Humanitarian Center
Ul. Borisa Galushkina 19A
129301 Moscow, Russia

MISSIONS AND DIANETICS CENTERS

BELARUS

Borisov Dianetics Center
222120 Borisov
2nd pereulok Turgeneva 19
Belarus

Dianetics Center of Minsk
220093 Minsk
Ul. Chilagze 31-89
Belarus

Scientology Mission of Mogilev
212011 Mogilev
Ul. Koroleva 37-2
Belarus

GEORGIA

Dianetics Mission of Tbilisi
380082 Tbilisi
Ul. Ushangi Chkheidze 8
Georgia

KAZAKHSTAN

Dianetics Center of Aktau
466200 Kazakhstan
Aktau 15-9-71
Kazakhstan

Dianetics Center of Almaty
480035 Almaty
8 Mikrorajon 4A
Kazakhstan

Dianetics Center of Astana
473000 Astana
Mikrorajon Tselinnij 5-15
Kazakhstan

Scientology Mission of Ekibastuz
638710 Ekibastuz
Ul. Satpajeva 8/16-4
Kazakhstan

Dianetics Center of Karaganda
470032 Karaganda
Erzhanova 10/2
Kazakhstan

Scientology Mission of Pavlodar
637000 Pavlodar
Ul. Lomova 135/1
Kazakhstan

Scientology Mission
  of Semipalatinsk
490035 Semipalatinsk
Ul. Pogranichnaya 44-11
Kazakhstan

Mission of Shymkent
486000 Shymkent
Ul. Bankelgina 33-55
Kazakhstan

Mission of Ust-Kamenogorsk
492000 Ust-Kamenogorsk
Ul. Proletarskaja 136-12
Kazakhstan

KYRGYZSTAN

Scientology Mission of Bishkek
Bishkek
Ul. Zhukeeva-Pudovkina 73
Kyrgyzstan

LATVIA
Scientology Mission of Riga
226000 Riga
A. Briana 9/1-15
Latvia

LITHUANIA
Scientology Mission of Vilnius
p.d. Nr. 42. LT 2000
Vilnius, Lithuania

MOLDOVA
Kishinev Dianetics Center
MD 2028, Kishinev
AB Box 1145
Moldova

RUSSIA
Scientology Mission of Arbat
103051 Moscow
Tzvetnoj Bulvar 26
Russia

Scientology Mission of Barnaul
656039 Barnaul
Ul. Malakhova 85-183, AB 507
Russia

Scientology Mission of Bryansk
242000 Bryansk
Ul. Fokina 3
Russia

Scientology Mission of Chelny
423800 Naberezhnije Chelny
AB 37
Russia

Scientology Mission
of Chelyabinsk
454138 Chelyabinsk
Komsomolskij proezd, 37 B-17
Russia

Dianetics Center of
Dimitrovgrad
433512 Ulyanovskaja Obl.
Dimitrovgrad
Prospect Dmitrova 14
AB Box 189
Russia

Mission of Dzerzhinsk
603167 N. Novgorod
Ul. Orenburskaja 7
Russia

Scientology Mission of
Ekaterinburg
620014 Ekaterinburg
Ul. Papanina 9
Russia

Scientology Mission of
Habarovsk
680014 Habarovsk
Pereulok Garazhnij 3-38
Russia

Dianetics Center of Ivanovo
153000 Ivanovo
Ul. 3rd Internationala 41-11
Russia

Scientology Mission of Izhevsk
426001 Izhevsk
AB 1903
Russia

Scientology Mission of
Kaliningrad
141070 Korolev
Moscow Region
Ul. Frunze 24-13
Russia

Scientology Mission of
Kalininskaya
195427 St. Petersburg
Ul. Vedeneeva 4-429
Russia

Dianetics Humanitarian Center
of Kaluga
248018 Kaluga
Ul. Marshala Zhukova 18
Russia

Scientology Mission of Kazan
420089 Kazan
Ul. Latyshskih Strelkov 33-171
Russia

Scientology Mission
of Kislovodsk
357746 Kislovodsk
Ul. Telmana 3-6
Russia

Scientology Mission
of Kostomuksha
186931 Kostomuksha
Ul. Lenina 8-27
Russia

Scientology Mission
of Krasnoselskaya
Leningrad Region
Gorod Gatchina
Ul. Novoproletarskaya 52-9
Russia

Dianetics Center of Krasnoyarsk
660077 Krasnoyarsk
Ul. Molokova 7-323
Russia

Scientology Mission of Kursk
305025 Kursk
Magistralny proezd 12-2
Russia

Scientology Mission of Kushva
624300 Kushva
Krasnoarmeiskaya 18-13
Russia

Scientology Mission
of Ligovskaya
193036 St. Petersburg
Ligovskij Prospect 33
Russia

Dianetics Center
of Magnitogorsk
455000 Magnitogorsk
AB Box 3008
Russia

Dianetics Center of Mitischi
141007 Moscovskaja Obl.
Mitischi
2-oj Shelkovsky proezd 5/1-62
Russia

Scientology Mission
of Moscovskaya
187110 Leningrad Region, Krishi
Bulvar Plavnitskoy 4-32
Russia

Scientology Mission of Moscow
109432 Moscow
2nd Juzhnoportovij proezd 27
Russia

Dianetics Center of Murmansk
183071 Murmansk
Prospect Svjazi 3
Russia

Mission of Naberezhnie Chelny
823427 Naberezhnie Chelny
Kamala 24-29
Russia

Dianetics Mission of Nazran
Ingushetija
Karabulak
Ul. Chkalova 38
Russia

Scientology Mission of
Nevinnomyssk
315714 Nevinnomyssk
Ul. Partizanskaya 11-122
Russia

Scientology Mission
of Nevskaja
188230 Leningrad Region, Luga
Ul. B. Zaretchnaja 74
Russia

Scientology Mission
of Nizhnekamsk
423570 Nizhnekamsk
Ul. 30 Let Pobedi 5
Russia

Dianetics Center
of Nizhny Novgorod
603167 Nizhny Novgorod
Ul. Orienburgskaja 7
Russia

Dianetics Center of
Novgorod
173001 Velikij Novgorod
Naberejnaja Reki Gzel 5
Russia

Scientology Mission
of Novokuznetsk
654079 Kemerovo Region
Novokuznetsk
Ul. Rostovskaja 13
Russia

Dianetics Center
of Novosibirsk
630087 Novosibirsk
AB 271
Russia

Scientology Mission
of Novy Urengoy
626718 Novy Urengoy
Ul. Youbeleynaya 1-41
Russia

Hubbard Humanitarian Center
of Obninsk
Moscow Region, Obninsk
Ul. Leshenko 6A-82
Russia

Hubbard Humanitarian Center
of Omsk I
644043 Omsk
AB Box 3768
Russia

Dianetics Center of Omsk II
644099 Omsk, Glavpochtamt
AB Box 333
Russia

Dianetics Center of Orenburg
460014 Orenburg
Ul. Tcheluskentsev 14
Russia

Scientology Mission of Oriol
302006 Oriol
Ul. Polikarpova 50-31, AB 255
Russia

Scientology Mission of Penza
440061 Penza
Ul. Tolstogo 8A
Penza, Russia

Dianetics Center of Perm
614002 Perm
Ul. Fontannaja 2A
Russia

Scientology Mission of
Perovskaya
111123 Moscow
Electronnij proezd 14-1
Russia

Scientology Mission of
Petrogradskaya
195176 St. Petersburg
Ul. Krasnodonskaja 19-9
Russia

Scientology Mission of
Kamchatka
683006 Petropavlovsk-
Kamchatskiy
Ul. Kavkazskaja 30/1-31
Russia

Scientology Mission of
Pushkinskaya
St. Petersburg, Pushkino
Ul. Shishkova 32/15-241
Russia

Dianetics Center of Samara
443041 Samara
AB 12746
Russia

Dianetics Center of Saratov
410600 Saratov
AB Box 1533
Russia

Scientology Mission of
Solnechnogorsk
141500 Solnechnogorsk-7
Ul. Podmoskovnaya 27-46
Russia

St. Petersburg
 Scientology Center II
192289 St. Petersburg
Ul. O. Dundicha 36-3-366
Russia

Scientology Mission
 of Severnaya
195176 St. Petersburg
Maneznij Per 17/15-12
Russia

Scientology Mission
 of Severomorsk
184600 Severomorsk
Ul. Dushenova 8/9-46
Russia

Dianetics Humanitarian
 Center of Surgut
628425 Surgut
Ul. Lermontova 6-1
Russia

Scientology Mission of Tambov
392032 Tambov Region
Pochtovoe Otdelenie 32, AB 12
Russia

Dianetics Humanitarian
 Center of Tolyatti
445050 Samarskaya Obl., Tolyatti
AB Box 14
Russia

Dianetics Center of Troitsk
142190 Troitsk
Sirenevaya 10-87
Russia

Scientology Mission of Tula
300000 Tula
Prospect Lenina 60-46
Russia

Dianetics Center of Ufa
450000 Ufa
Ul. Zemtsova 70
Russia

Scientology Mission of Ulan-Ude
670009 Ulan-Ude
Ul. Nevskaya 11
Buryatia, Russia

Scientology Mission of Uljanovsk
432072 Uljanovsk
Ul. Zheleznodorozhnaja 14-23
Russia

Scientology Mission
 of Vladivostok
690001 Vladivostok
Borisenko 33-10
Russia

Dianetics Humanitarian
 Center of Volgograd
400075 Volgograd
Ul. Kirova 112-63
Russia

Scientology Mission of Voronezh
394051 Voronezh
Ul. Domostroitelej 2-34
Russia

Scientology Mission
 of Zheleznogorsk
662971 Zheleznogorsk
Ul. Severnaja 315
AB 668
Russia

UKRAINE

Hubbard Humanitarian Center
 of Harkov
Harkov
Ul. Kotlova 83
Dom Nauki i Tekhniki, AB 53
Ukraine

Scientology Mission
 of Kremenchug
Kremenchug
Ul. 60 Let Octiabria 45-24
Ukraine

Scientology Mission
of Melitopol
Melitopol
Ul. Grizodubovoj 42-118
Ukraine

Scientology Mission of Nikolayev
54056 Nikolayev
Ul. Artelerijskaja 18, AB 98
Ukraine

Dianetics Center of Uzhgorod
88000 Uzhgorod
Ul. Dobrianskogo 10-9
Ukraine

UNITED KINGDOM

Scientology Missions
International
United Kingdom Office
Saint Hill Manor
East Grinstead
West Sussex, England
RH19 4JY

MISSIONS AND DIANETICS CENTERS

Dianetics and Scientology
Mission of Bournemouth Ltd
42 High Street
Poole, Dorset, England
BH15 1BT

Church of Scientology
Mission of Hove Ltd
59A Coleridge Street
Hove, East Sussex, England
BN3 5AB

HONG KONG

Church of Scientology
Mission of Hong Kong
Flat E, 7/F, Tower 8
Laguna Verde
Hung Hom, Kowloon
Central, Hong Kong

INDIA

Mysore Mission
Chamundi Footstep Road
JSS ashram
Mysore, Larna 57004
India

Dianetics Center
of Ambala Cantt
6352 Punjabi Mohalla
Ambala Cantt 133001
India

Dianetics Center
of Calcutta
P404/2 Hemanta
Mukhopadhyay Sarani
Calcutta 700029
India

IRELAND

Church of Scientology
Mission of Dublin Ltd
62/63 Middle Abbey Street
Dublin 1, Ireland

JAPAN

Church of Scientology
Dianetics Centre Akasaka
Akasaka-dori 50 Building, 5-5-11
Akasaka Minato-ku
Tokyo, Japan

LATIN AMERICA

Scientology Missions
International
Latin American Office
Puebla 31, Colonia Roma
CP 06700 Mexico, D.F.

MISSIONS AND DIANETICS CENTERS

COLOMBIA

Asociación Dianética
Bogotá Norte
Avenida 13, No. 104-91
Bogotá, Colombia

Fundación para el
Mejoramiento de la Vida
Calle 70A, No. 12-38
Bogotá, Colombia

Iglesia de Cienciología
Misión de Medellín
Carrera 13, No. 19-23
La Ceja, Antioquia, Colombia

CHILE

Centro de Tecnología Hubbard
Jorge Washington, No. 338
Santiago de Chile, Chile

Centro Hubbard
Misión de Chile
Nuncio Laghi, 6558
La Reina, Santiago, Chile

COSTA RICA

Instituto Tecnológico
de Dianética
PO Box 3010
1150 San José
Costa Rica

DOMINICAN REPUBLIC

Dianética Santo Domingo
Condominio Ambar Plaza II
Bloque II, Apto. 302
Avenida Núñez de Cáceres Esq.
Sarasota
Santo Domingo
Dominican Republic

ECUADOR

Iglesia de Cienciología
Misión de Guayaquil
Avenida Fco. de Orellana
No. 218
Guayaquil, Ecuador

GUATEMALA

Asociación de Cienciología
Aplicada Dianética
de Guatemala
21 Avenida "A," 32-28
Zona 5, Guatemala

MEXICO

Centro de Dianética Hubbard
de Aguascalientes A.C.
Hamburgo, No. 127
Fraccionamiento del Valle 1A Sec.
C.P. 20080 Aguascalientes, Ags.
Mexico

Instituto de Filosofía
Aplicada de Bajío
Boulevard Adolfo López Mateos
507 Oriente
Zona Centro Entre Libertad y
República
Leon Gto.
C.P. 37000, Mexico

Mission Chihuahua
Calle Septima 501-A
Rancheria Juarez-Chihuahua
Chihuahua, Mexico

Centro Hubbard de Dianética
Tecamachalco
#314 Prsdo. Norte
Lomas de Chapultepec
Mexico, D.F. Mexico

Instituto de Dianética
Monterrey A.C.
Tulancingo, 1262, Col. Mitras
Monterrey
N.L., Mexico

Mission of Mexicali
Au. plan de Acatempan
#1635 Fracc. La Rivera
Mexicali, BC.
C.P. 21269, Mexico

Misión de Satelite
Calle Alamo, #93-3er Piso –
Local B
Santa Monica, Tlalnepantla
Edo. de Mexico, 54040
Mexico

Misión de Tijuana
Calle Balboa, #5284
Lomas Hipódromo
Tijuana B.C.
C.P. 22480 Mexico

Misión de Valle
Juárez, 139
San Pedro Garza García
N.L. Monterrey, 66230 Mexico

PAKISTAN

Dianetics Center
A-3 Royal Avenue
(opposite Urdu College
 Block 13C)
Gulshan-E-Iqbal
Karachi, Pakistan

TAIWAN

Scientology Missions
 International
Taiwan Office
2F, No. 65, Sec. 4
Ming-Shung East Road
Taipei, Taiwan

MISSIONS AND DIANETICS CENTERS

Church of Scientology
Mission of Capital
2F No. 28, Lane 63
Liao-Ning Street
Taipei, Taiwan

Church of Scientology
Mission of Kaohsiung
No. 216, Fu-Jen Road
Ling-Ya District
Kaohsiung, Taiwan

Church of Scientology
Mission of Pingtung
No. 206, Pang-Chiu Road
Pingtung, Taiwan

Church of Scientology
Mission of Taichung
No. 82-2 Wu-Chuan-5th Street
Taichung, Taiwan

Church of Scientology
Mission of Tainan
3F, No. 70, Ching-Nien Road
Tainan, Taiwan

Church of Scientology
Mission of Taipei
No. 2, Lane 59, Sec. 2
Sung-Chang North Road
Taipei, Taiwan

THAILAND

Church of Scientology
Mission of Bangkok
Room B1, 2F, 339 Soi Pipat
Bangrak
Bangkok, Thailand 10500

TO OBTAIN ANY BOOKS OR CASSETTES BY L. RON HUBBARD WHICH ARE NOT AVAILABLE AT YOUR LOCAL ORGANIZATION, CONTACT ANY OF THE FOLLOWING PUBLICATIONS ORGANIZATIONS WORLDWIDE:

BRIDGE PUBLICATIONS, INC.
4751 Fountain Avenue
Los Angeles, California 90029
www.bridgepub.com

Rua Alfonso Celso 115
Vila Mariana São Paulo, SP
04119-000 Brazil

CONTINENTAL PUBLICATIONS
LIAISON OFFICE
696 Yonge Street
Toronto, Ontario
Canada M4Y 2A7

NEW ERA PUBLICATIONS
INTERNATIONAL ApS
Store Kongensgade 53
1264 Copenhagen K
Denmark
www.newerapublications.com

ERA DINÁMICA EDITORES,
S.A. DE C.V.
Pablo Ucello #16
Colonia C.D. de los Deportes
Mexico, D.F.

NEW ERA PUBLICATIONS
UK LTD
Saint Hill Manor
East Grinstead, West Sussex
England RH19 4JY

NEW ERA PUBLICATIONS
AUSTRALIA PTY LTD
Level 1, 61–65 Wentworth
Avenue
Surry Hills, New South Wales
Australia 2000

CONTINENTAL PUBLICATIONS
PTY LTD
6th Floor, Budget House
130 Main Street
Johannesburg 2001
South Africa

NEW ERA PUBLICATIONS
ITALIA S.R.L.
Via Cadorna, 61
20090 Vimodrone (MI), Italy

NEW ERA PUBLICATIONS
DEUTSCHLAND GMBH
Hittfelder Kirchweg 5A
21220 Seevetal-Maschen
Germany

NEW ERA PUBLICATIONS
FRANCE E.U.R.L.
14, rue des Moulins
75001 Paris, France

NUEVA ERA DINÁMICA, S.A.
C/ Montera 20, 1° dcha.
28013 Madrid, Spain

NEW ERA PUBLICATIONS
JAPAN, INC.
Sakai SS bldg 2F, 4-38-15
Higashi-Ikebukuro
Toshima-ku, Tokyo, Japan 170-0013

NEW ERA PUBLICATIONS GROUP
Str. Kasatkina 16, Building 1
129301 Moscow, Russia

NEW ERA PUBLICATIONS
CENTRAL EUROPEAN OFFICE
1438 Budapest
Pf. 351
Hungary

"*I am always happy to hear from my readers.*"

L. Ron Hubbard

THESE WERE THE WORDS of L. Ron Hubbard, who was always very interested in hearing from his friends and readers. He made a point of staying in communication with everyone he came in contact with over his more than fifty-year career as a professional writer, and he had thousands of fans and friends that he corresponded with all over the world.

The author's representatives, Author Services, Inc., wish to continue this tradition and welcome letters and comments from you, his readers, both old and new.

Additionally, they will be happy to send you information on anything you would like to know about L. Ron Hubbard, his extraordinary life and accomplishments and the vast number of books he has written.

Any message addressed to the Author's Affairs Director at Author Services, Inc., will be given prompt and full attention.

Author Services, Inc.

7051 HOLLYWOOD BOULEVARD
HOLLYWOOD, CALIFORNIA 90028, USA

authoraffairs@authorservicesinc.com

ABOUT
THE
AUTHOR

ABOUT
THE AUTHOR

AUTHOR, PHILOSOPHER, HUMANITARIAN—L. Ron Hubbard is one of the most acclaimed figures of the modern age. His works have inspired millions, primarily because they provide the answers to the most profound questions of human existence—and do so in ways all people can understand.

As Ron said, "One doesn't learn about life sitting in an ivory tower, thinking about it. One learns about life by being part of it." And that is how he lived.

His quest began at a very early age. By the time he was eight years old, he was already well on his way to being a seasoned traveler and his adventures included then rare voyages to China, Japan and other points in the Orient and South Pacific. In all, he traversed a quarter of a million miles by the age of nineteen. In the course of his travels he became closely acquainted with twenty-one different races and cultures in all parts of the world.

In the fall of 1930, Ron pursued studies of mathematics and engineering at George Washington University, attending one of the first American classes on nuclear physics. Examination of these subjects brought him to the realization that neither the East nor the West contained the full answer to the problems of existence, despite all of mankind's advances in the physical sciences. He observed the mental "technologies" which did exist—psychology and psychiatry—to be barbaric, false subjects and no more workable than the inhuman methods of primitive witch doctors. Ron decided to shoulder the responsibility of filling the gap, knowing man needed to step far beyond the materialistic world in which he was embroiled.

Much of his early research was financed by his career as a fiction writer. He became one of the most highly demanded authors of the golden age of popular adventure and science fiction writing during the '30s and '40s—interrupted only by his service in the US Navy during World War II.

Partially disabled at the end of the war and recuperating in Oak Knoll Naval Hospital in Oakland, California, Ron applied what he had discovered as a result of his research into the mind to not only recover fully from his own injuries but also to help others to regain the health they lost through the ravages of war. He engaged in a study of the endocrine system and the effect of the mind on the body's ability to absorb and use nutrients which resulted in the brand-new discovery that structure does not monitor function, as medicine believed, but the reverse was true: function (or life) monitors structure.

In 1947, Ron detailed his discoveries in a manuscript which circulated amongst his friends, who copied it and passed it on to others. (This manuscript was formally published in 1951 as *Dianetics: The Original Thesis* and later republished as *The Dynamics of Life*.) Floods of inquiries were generated by this material; in response, Ron wrote a comprehensive text on the subject—*Dianetics: The Modern Science of Mental Health*.

Published on May 9, 1950, *Dianetics: The Modern Science of Mental Health* made his revolutionary ideas broadly available for the first time. Public interest spread like wildfire and the book shot to the top of the *New York Times* bestseller list and remained there week after week. More than 750 Dianetics study groups sprang up coast to coast within a few months of its publication, while newspaper headlines proclaimed: "Dianetics Takes US by Storm."

After the success of *Dianetics,* demand from the public accelerated and Ron conducted numerous lecture tours to packed halls throughout the country—all the while relentlessly continuing his research. Through the '50s, he wrote six more books as he continued to make breakthrough after breakthrough, forming the very fundamentals leading to the development of Scientology, the first workable technology for the improvement of all aspects of life.

Ron's unrelenting pursuit of more refined technology whereby man might increase awareness and lead a happier, more productive life led him to research all barriers to spiritual gains. He found that spiritual advancement came to a standstill under the effect of drugs, not to mention the suppression of a culture itself under drug-related crime.

"Drugs can apparently change the attitude of a person from his original personality to one secretly harboring hostilities and hatreds he does not permit to show on the surface," wrote Ron. "While this may not hold true in all cases, it does establish a link between drugs and increasing difficulties with crime, production and the modern breakdown of social and industrial culture."

Determined to overcome the scourge of drugs and open the gates to spiritual gain for all, Ron conducted extensive studies in the fields of vitamins, minerals and nutrition. These studies paved the way to startling discoveries, including methodology which saved drug addicts from painful and dangerous withdrawal symptoms. Ron was also the first to discover that residues from drugs and other toxins lodge in the tissues of the body and can adversely continue to affect one for years, perhaps decades after. From this and further research into the devastating consequences of accumulated drugs and toxins in the body, he developed and released the Purification program in 1979.

Continuing his quest to help man overcome the obstacles to living, Ron carried on his research and writing through 1985, amassing an enormous volume of material. Totaling over 60 million words—recorded in books, manuscripts and taped lectures—these works are studied and applied daily in hundreds of Scientology churches, missions and organizations around the world.

With his research fully completed and codified, L. Ron Hubbard departed his body on 24 January 1986. His legacy lives on, however, opening the way for a prosperous and flourishing life for millions by bringing them understanding and freedom.

Today there is a pathway for anyone to travel to attain full spiritual freedom. The entrance is wide and the route is sure. We have L. Ron Hubbard to acknowledge as the one who made it all possible.

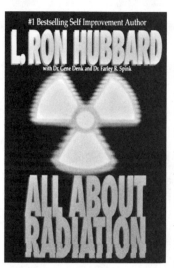

DRUGS, TOXINS & RADIATION DESTROY YOUR LIFE.

Get rid of them!

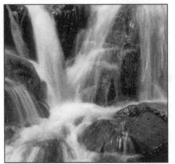

The filthy effects of toxic residues and radiation can send your whole life crashing. These substances put you in a condition which not only destroys your physical health, but prevents any stable advancement in mental or spiritual well-being.

Like a fresh stream of crystal clear water, the Scientology Purification Program gets rid of the devastating effects of drugs, toxins and radiation so they no longer block your clear thinking and enthusiasm for life. This breakthrough discovery by L. Ron Hubbard has helped hundreds of thousands lead happy, more perceptive and aware lives.

YOU NEED THIS PROGRAM!

Do the Scientology Purification Program

Contact the Registrar at your local Church of Scientology to sign up for the Purification Program.

See page 217 for the location of the church nearest you.

www.clearbodyclearmind.com